How to Respond in a Pandemic

Sara Miller McCune founded SAGE Publishing in 1965 to support the dissemination of usable knowledge and educate a global community. SAGE publishes more than 1000 journals and over 800 new books each year, spanning a wide range of subject areas. Our growing selection of library products includes archives, data, case studies and video. SAGE remains majority owned by our founder and after her lifetime will become owned by a charitable trust that secures the company's continued independence.

Los Angeles | London | New Delhi | Singapore | Washington DC | Melbourne

How to Respond in a Pandemic

25 Ideas From 25 Disciplines of Study

Joan Ferrante

Northern Kentucky University

Chris Caldeira

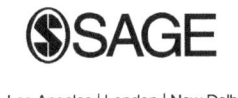

Los Angeles | London | New Delhi
Singapore | Washington DC | Melbourne

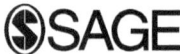

FOR INFORMATION:

SAGE Publications, Inc.
2455 Teller Road
Thousand Oaks, California 91320
E-mail: order@sagepub.com

SAGE Publications Ltd.
1 Oliver's Yard
55 City Road
London, EC1Y 1SP
United Kingdom

SAGE Publications India Pvt. Ltd.
B 1/I 1 Mohan Cooperative Industrial Area
Mathura Road, New Delhi 110 044
India

SAGE Publications Asia-Pacific Pte. Ltd.
18 Cross Street #10-10/11/12
China Square Central
Singapore 048423

Library of Congress Control Number: 2020942008

ISBN 978-1-0718-3595-1 (pbk) | 978-10718-3596-8 (epub) | 978-1-0718-3597-5 (epub)

Acquisitions Editor: Jeff Lasser
Editorial Assistant: Tiara Beatty
Production Editor: Tracy Buyan
Typesetter: Hurix Digital
Proofreader: Barbara Coster
Cover Designer: Rose Storey
Marketing Manager: Jennifer Jones

20 21 22 23 24 10 9 8 7 6 5 4 3 2 1

Contents

Annotated Contents

Sociology
Know That Things Are Not What They Seem
Joan Ferrante and Chris Caldeira
The sociological lens compels us to look below the surface to see that things are not what they seem. We can understand the world in new ways if we move beyond our immediate social circles to take in others' perspectives. Similarly, sociology does not stand alone; it partners with other disciplines to strengthen and deliver meaningful and relevant analyses, especially in times of crisis.

Anthropology
Connect and Reconnect With Food
Sharyn Jones
Anthropologists who study food look at the fascinating relationship between humans and what they eat. When food systems break down, communities and civilizations collapse. And in troubling times, food provides a mode of connecting and reconnecting with our humanity, our community, and the Earth.

Biology
Look to Science for Answers
Emina Atikovic
In a pandemic, biologists can provide insight into critical questions such as "How is this virus different from others?" and "Why does soap and water kill the virus?" Biologists can also offer commentary about whether the film *Contagion* accurately depicts the way a pandemic plays out (in some ways it's accurate, in other ways not).

Clinical Counseling
Work to Become Resilient
Isabella Zembrodt
The discipline of counseling provides frames for supporting resilience. Talking through unresolved issues helps us unpack previous experiences that stand in the way of making constructive responses. In the process, we are able to reimagine a new personal narrative and gain an empowering perspective.

Community Engagement
Engage in New Ways
Mark Neikirk
This crisis has severely compromised the in-person, experiential component of student community engagement projects. As one illustration, student

philanthropy projects were disrupted when universities across the country transitioned to all online learning. Students were forced to adapt, be flexible, and innovate to carry out their valuable work. There is no lesson more important than learning to change strategies midstream and continue moving forward.

Creative Writing
Slow Down, Pause, Reflect
Kelly Moffett

When our minds are rushing forward in a haze of anxiety, confusion, and overinformation, engaging with poetry delivers an experience of slowing down. It facilitates a state of calm, self-expression, and insight.

Critical White Studies
Grasp the Deeper Meaning of Social Distancing
Joan Ferrante and Prince Brown Jr., with India Hackle

Mandating physical space between people is not a new practice in the United States. For over 400 years, governments at all levels enforced physical distancing along racial lines. It is important to grasp the deeper meaning and relevance of this history and how it still affects our lives today.

Cultural Studies
Change the Story, Change What Is Possible
John Alberti

Stories are how we make sense of what is happening in the world and in our daily lives. When we talk about getting "back to normal" after the coronavirus pandemic, we are really talking about returning to a familiar story that used to define reality for us. Crises present opportunities to create new stories. Cultural studies reminds us that these stories are ours to create and share together.

Developmental Mathematics
Embrace the Math You Thought You Would Never Need
Elizabeth McMillan-McCartney

Math is essential for understanding the impact of this novel coronavirus and evaluating our responses to it. You would be surprised at how basic math and algebra (adding, subtracting, multiplying, and dividing) allow you to think in sophisticated ways about an event that is affecting us all.

English Literature
Read, Write, Make Meaning
Robert K. Wallace

Enforced periods of social distancing and isolation do not diminish our need to make meaning, and indeed, may enhance it. Reading autobiographies such as the *Narrative of the Life of Frederick Douglass, an American Slave* allows us to see how someone living through a crisis can write about it. The process of writing also helps us navigate a difficult time or come to a new understanding.

Environmental Sociology
Don't Blame the Bats
Jaime McCauley

The story of how the COVID-19 pandemic came to be ultimately has little to do with bats in China. While nonhuman animals may play a role in disease transmission, human activity is the driving force. We must look at how environmental degradation has forced animals into human-occupied spaces.

Film Studies
See the Predictability in the Chaos of Pandemics
Tom Zaniello

Epidemic cinema gives us imagery and narratives that shape the public's perception of pandemics and infectious diseases—of how they came to be and how they move through populations. The films focus on all that can go wrong. The mayhem depicted in these films mirrors the chaos of real pandemics, allowing us to see some predictability in the events that unfold in such crises.

Health Economics
Behave as if You Are Contagious
Linda Dynan

To get through this health care crisis, everyone must participate in collective action aimed at reducing transmission. Ironically, even though social distancing comes at a high personal and economic cost, it is necessary for economic survival. Think of social distancing as an investment—in your own and others' health, in the economy, and in the health care system.

History
Discover a Blueprint to See a Way Out
William Landon

When historians are asked to comment on this current crisis, they direct us to look at previous pandemics and how humanity responded to and overcame them. By looking to the past, we can learn which actions and treatments were most effective. Knowing the past helps us gain our bearings as we navigate tumultuous waters.

Informatics
Know How Your Information Is Being Shared
Kevin Kirby

In a time of crisis, information surges. The emergence of contact-tracing apps has brought into focus the tension between sharing and hiding information, between what we as individuals want to keep private and what we want to make public. Before signing on with any apps, we must consider who is consuming our information, and to what end.

Mathematics
Turn to Mathematics to Know How We Are Doing
Phil McCartney

Mathematics is about thinking through complex questions for which answers are not readily knowable. In this paper, we look at how mathematicians employ thought experiments to think through complex questions about how we are doing and where we are heading in this pandemic.

Music
Support the Artists You Turn to in Times of Crisis
Jason Vest

We turn to music for comfort because it has a powerful effect on our well-being, intellect, and ability to deal with grief and trauma. Anytime we freely consume music, we must remind ourselves to find ways to support the artists who create it.

Organizational Leadership
Understand That Crises Can Be Managed
Nana Arthur-Mensah

In times of crisis, we turn to leaders for answers and guidance. Effective leaders know there are phases in a crisis and that each phase requires a specific set of skills. They know, too, that these skills can be learned, and they take the necessary steps to acquire them.

Philosophy
Stand Up for the Marginalized and Vulnerable
Yaw A. Frimpong-Mansoh

Philosophers take interest in the ethics underlying the decisions of policy makers and ordinary citizens, especially during a crisis. One notable frame for evaluating such decisions is egalitarian ethics, which is concerned with justice and equality, especially for the marginalized and the vulnerable.

Political Science
Join Together in an Age of Apart
Ryan Salzman

In the U.S. democratic system, "the people" form groups, which both support and limit the power of elected leaders. While there have been impressively organized protests throughout this pandemic, the ability to associate face-to-face in group settings has been severely compromised. We must take action to reestablish the force of joining together, even if associating takes new forms.

Psychological Science
Imagine How the Pandemic Affects Everyone Across the Lifespan
Allyson S. Graf

This pandemic has altered the path of everyone's life, albeit in different ways. When we consider lifespan principles, we understand what people in all age groups are going through. We are all capable of change in a crisis, and understanding this can help us confront the ambiguity around the virus as we move along our life path.

School Counseling
Keep Looking for the Students Who Have Not Connected
Donita Jackson

When the threat of COVID-19 put schools in lockdown, counselors found themselves in a new role—tracking down students who could not or did not connect virtually. Counselors, trained to understand that there are always reasons for absenteeism, make it their mission to find ways to remove barriers to connecting. This is not solely a responsibility of counselors. Students, too, can take notice of peers who are not connecting and reach out with understanding.

Trauma Studies
Learn How Trauma Impacts Us
La Shanda Sugg

In times of personal and societal crisis, human survival responses such as flock, flight-fight, freeze, and faint are activated. If we can learn to identify our reactions and how past experiences motivate them, we can more skillfully manage our responses and better understand ourselves and others.

Visual Arts
Visualize Social Issues
Robert Del Tredici

Sometimes the process used in a photography project to document one complex, challenging topic may shed light on a process for documenting a quite different topic. Photographs and interviews documenting the effects of radioactivity released by the mass production of nuclear weapons and commercial nuclear reactors can act as a road map for tracking the effects of the COVID-19 pandemic.

World Languages
Learn How Another Culture Responds to Crises
Bo-Kyung Kim Kirby

Cultural values and assumptions shape response to any crisis. To illustrate, this paper considers one case: South Korea's response to COVID-19. We can see how cultural assumptions, including those revealed in the Korean language, supported social distancing, mask wearing, and contact tracing, ultimately catapulting it as a model among countries for controlling the spread of the virus.

Preface

The COVID-19 pandemic has altered people's lives and interactions in drastic ways, casting a long shadow over an uncertain future. It has exposed deeply rooted inequalities that affect who gets sick, who can succeed in school, and who becomes unemployed. Even if we believe our lives have not changed much,[1] it is impossible to extract ourselves from the effects this pandemic has had on our communities, country, and planet.

By now, most of us know the guidelines for how to prevent the spread of this virus (whether we are following them or not), but we lack guidelines for how to weather the social and personal upheavals. When the pandemic hit, the 17.8 million students enrolled in colleges and universities across the United States likely looked to their peers and instructors for help with processing the crisis—to make some sense of all that was happening to them and around them. In choosing their courses and deciding on majors, they had signed on to ways of seeing the world, and they wanted to know how those perspectives held up now. If we consider the other 139 million people[2] who have completed college degrees or taken at least one college course at some stage of life, the meaning-making lure of higher education is undeniable.

The inspiration for *How to Respond in a Pandemic: 25 Ideas From 25 Disciplines of Study* came as decisions to lock down campuses were made and many students suddenly lost access to food, housing, the Internet, and other resources.[3] In the midst of these changes and stresses we asked: What can our discipline of sociology offer? Then our thoughts extended to, What can other disciplines offer?

In this time of crisis, we felt it was important for the academic disciplines to respond. We aimed to incorporate a diversity of perspectives and to transcend disciplinary boundaries. Out of this felt urgency, the idea for this book was born. We issued invitations to experts working at, or connected to, Northern Kentucky University to submit a paper of three to five pages focusing on one idea that serves as one voice from their discipline.[4] Our goal was to recruit 25 authors from 25 different areas of study.[5] And we did. The collection is one campus's response, but it is also a response from higher education.

Along the way—from March 19 (the start date) to July 2 (the date this book went into production)—these 25 authors wrestled with difficult questions. How will we address the COVID-19 pandemic and the Black Lives Matter movement that erupted within it? How do we revamp our ideas in light of these two events? What do we say, for example, to students majoring in the arts whose opportunities to perform have been severely limited? What do we say to students who may be reevaluating or reconfirming their career choice? And what about students playing sports who do not know when they will compete again, or if they do, wonder if events or seasons will all be called off another time? What do we say about the cultural tensions that this pandemic has intensified? Will our ideas matter to students whose anxieties and fears interfere with their learning? So many questions, but they must be asked and answered.

The Process

While each idea paper is unique and discipline inspired, they are guided by a collaborative goal: to make a coherent response to the crises we face. Readers will notice that each idea paper is short and concise. Each title is a call to action. Within the paper, the author defines the discipline and focuses on one idea that the discipline can offer.

The authors are writing with readers in mind. They did not give in to the fears that typically haunt them when they write for scholarly journals. That is, they resisted the urge to write defensively as they might normally do to avoid harshly issued critiques from those reviewers who have traumatized us all.[6] When authors write defensively, they overcite and include unnecessary asides and caveats, hoping to ward off the critics. But in their bios, our authors included only the most essential information and their core credentials (even though they all could boast of many accomplishments). Instead, their bios focus on why they trust in the idea they present.

The authors agreed to be part of an unconventional review and editorial process, in which they did the hard work of creating a draft—the most difficult part of writing—which included settling on the idea and working through how to best present it. Then each of the 11 reviewers, including professors, current students, recent graduates, and community stakeholders, read each paper. Five editors—the two editors of this collection, two reader advocate editors, and a trusted copy editor—reviewed the writing, line by line, word for word. The authors considered the critiques and revised or accepted revisions accordingly, but they always had the last word.

The authors also recognized that they bring a lifetime of learning to what they write, while students are new to these ideas and come from various disciplines. So, in an effort to present their ideas clearly to all readers, the authors embraced the feedback of thoughtful reviewers and editors, who pointed out when they were confused or in need of more (or less) explanation. The number of hours put into each of the resulting idea papers is surprising.[7] (For more on this process, see the reader advocate editors' preface that follows.)

F. Scott Fitzgerald wrote, "The loneliest moment in someone's life is when they are watching their whole world fall apart, and all they can do is stare blankly."[8] Unlike those described in Fitzgerald's assertion, our authors were not staring blankly into space—they were writing their idea with both a twist and clarity that you cannot find searching online.

While each discipline has a distinct focus, you will notice that the disciplines also have much in common and often draw from one another. For example, you will see a biologist writing about a film also discussed in the film studies paper. You will read about the call for people to rewrite their narrative in the clinical counseling paper and the call for groups and society to create new stories in the cultural studies paper. And few disciplines can do without thought-driven mathematical calculations in discussing the pandemic.

We thank each contributor who took on this project with the goal of making a unified response to the crisis. Taken together, these 25 idea papers offer the readers some guidance for how to make sense of and take action in times of crisis. We also thank our team of reviewers, reader advocates, and copy editor: Angela Lackey (Alternative Learning Center Facilitator, Cincinnati Public Schools), Simon Gores (Biology major), India Hackle (International Studies and English, class of 2020, graduate student MFA Creative Writing Program at Cornell University, Reader Advocate Co-Editor), Lynnissa Hillman (Sociology Instructor), Kirsten Hurst (Creative Writing, Reader Advocate Co-editor), Dana Johnson (MS, Molecular & Cellular Physiology) Mariah Jones (English major, class of 2020), Sherman Parnell (Visual Arts, class of 2020), Ryan Salzman (Associate Professor of Political Science), La Shanda Sugg (Trauma Therapist and Consultant, the Mourning the Creation of Racial Categories Project). Finally, we thank Michele Sordi (Sr. Vice President and Head of U.S. College at SAGE) and Jeff Lasser (Sociology Publisher, SAGE) for believing in this project.

The Need for Reader Advocates

●●●

This collection of 25 ideas from 25 disciplines of study is unique in that it presents what higher education can offer in a pandemic—or any crisis, for that matter. This edited volume is also unique because it breaks from a centuries-old model that has been referred to as "sage on the stage." In that model, the sage—an all-knowing author—imparts knowledge to students. The sage on the stage can be likened to an expert lecturing to students standing behind a closed door. The sage knows that students are on the other side, but it does not matter who they are or what they are thinking.

Sages have no incentive to open the door to ask if their ideas are relevant and resonate. They do not consider how the students are experiencing their words. And sages do not take the time to gauge whether their message inspires students to think, do, or live differently.

This book project broke from the traditional sage-on-the stage model. A team of reader advocates—students, recent college graduates, and professors—was assembled to provide feedback about each idea paper. As reader advocates, we focused on places in the author's writing that tripped us up. We marked areas where we struggled with inconsistencies, lost concentration, and encountered ideas that (while interesting) interrupted the flow. If we found an area that made us pause in confusion, we assumed other readers would have the same reaction. We also noted where the writing drew us in and made us want to know more. Finally, we imagined how we might take in the writing if we were not us—if we were younger or older, held different jobs, or came from different communities.

Why bring in a team of reader advocates? Because reading is hard work, and the writing should ease that work, not make it more difficult. After all, reading is a physically, emotionally, and mentally demanding activity.[1] It takes work just to get the body to sit still long enough to focus on and get through the text. But sitting still is not enough; readers also have to turn off distracting thoughts that interfere with the words, sentences, and paragraphs before them. The mind interrupts to wonder if the stove is turned off, to check a text message, or to pet the cat or dog. It interrupts to tell you the room is too hot, too cold, and the chair too uncomfortable. And these are just a few of the routine concerns. What about the effort it takes to read in times of a pandemic? The mind races with thoughts about getting to the store before the shelves empty, or losing a job, or connecting with loved ones, especially if they are sick or dying.

Once the mind is cleared—as well as it can be—then comes the work of applying knowledge and life experiences to the text. Readers are engaged with the text when they are able to reconstruct its ideas in ways that are personally meaningful and when the words prompt them to rethink, reframe, or verify what they already know and have experienced. They engage not only with the author but also with ideas bigger than the self. This type of personal connection is what makes the reading experience a meaningful one.

When the 25 authors signed on to write idea papers for this collection, not only did they agree to do the hard work of writing, they also agreed to put their egos aside and hear what readers think, where they get lost, and when they feel spoken to (or ignored). That our authors welcomed and accepted feedback is a clear sign that they do not care to be the sage on the stage. Rather than assuming that something is wrong with readers who cannot follow their writing, the authors were committed to meeting readers where they are. By embracing the team-oriented mindset that this review process requires, these authors opened the door and spoke with the people—the reader advocates—behind it.

Readers will bring to these pages varied fears and concerns about their future, as well as worries about the relevance of education. They are unsure of what this new "normal" will bring and what they will lose to make room for it. Still, in the face of every major crisis, people forge ahead. Empathy is at the heart of this collection of idea papers. We feel it in the collaborative spirit between a team of 25 authors and 11 reader advocates banding together to create a readable guide for how to respond in a crisis.

India Hackle and Kirsten Hurst
Reader Advocate Editors

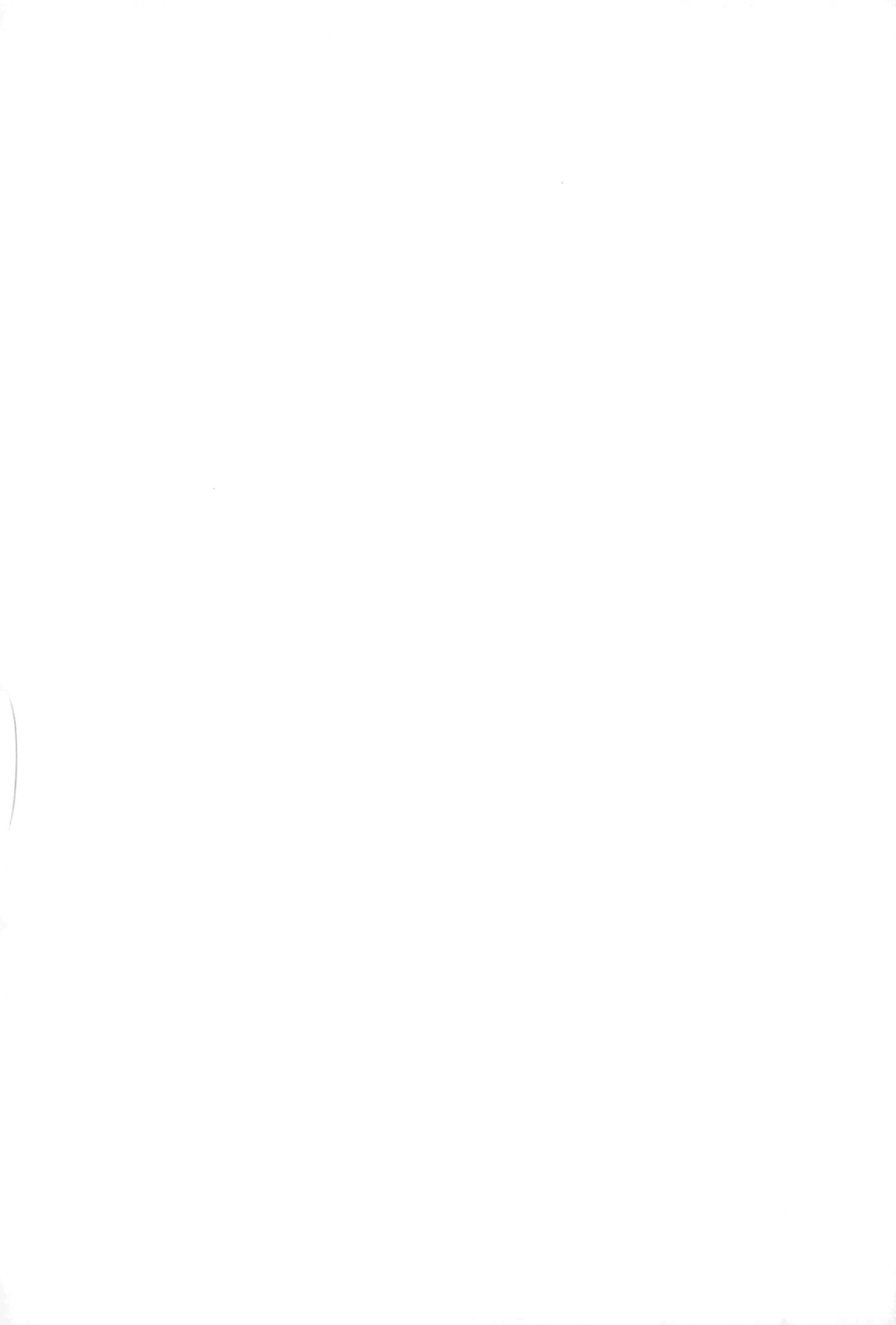

Know That Things Are Not What They Seem

Joan Ferrante and Chris Caldeira

Sociology

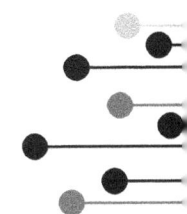

Sociology is the study of social forces that shape human lives. To illustrate this idea, imagine a group of sociologists walking down the streets of your neighborhood in the wake of the COVID-19 pandemic. They need to understand why things look the way they do. They pay attention to the businesses that closed permanently as a result of the lockdown. They notice if a grocery store is in the heart of the neighborhood or miles away. They observe the racial composition of the people walking or driving by. Sociologists look at the effects of COVID-19, the location of grocery stores, and racial composition as immediate forces that affect your neighborhood and the people who live there.[1]

Sociologists are not content to take at face value what they see. The discipline trains and even compels them to look below the surface. Sociologists want to be invited inside homes and buildings to see how people live. They welcome a tour of basements and attics, living rooms and closets, to learn about what is hidden from view. Sociologists leave their comfort zones to talk with people and observe them as they work, interact, and otherwise live their lives. They do not let a setting's reputation as dangerous, or even ordinary, interfere with their need to learn. Sociologists do not seek to exploit or disgrace. Rather, they are interested in getting to know people in the context of their communities. The way sociologists go about studying social forces can be summed up with the motto "Things are not what they seem."[2]

Sociologists know that people's options for responding to the COVID-19 pandemic expand or constrict depending on the resources they hold (e.g., income, occupation, support system) and can draw upon[3] (savings accounts, inheritance, home equity, social connections). They also know that the ways in which people think about the pandemic depends on who they most closely interact with—family, friends, and acquaintances. If nurses or doctors are in your social circle, the strain on hospitals is an urgent topic of conversation. If you know a delivery driver, you hear about pressures to deliver an avalanche of packages under tight deadlines. If many around you are unemployed, how to survive without money weighs on every conversation. The point is that how we experience the pandemic is constrained by who we interact with.

So how do we break free from these constraints? The discipline of sociology presents us with useful concepts that open our eyes beyond what we can glean from our immediate social contacts. One concept is *anticipated versus unanticipated consequences*.[4] In the context of the COVID-19 crisis, this concept alerts us to the countless ways people experience and respond to the new coronavirus—ways that may be different from our own.

The word *anticipated* prompts us to look for responses to the pandemic that we can easily predict. When businesses close, we expect that millions of people will lose jobs and that low-wage workers will be the hardest hit. We can anticipate an underground economy of hairstylists and personal trainers meeting clients in their homes. With social distancing, we expect more loneliness and solitary activities. But we also expect that people will find new ways to congregate.

The word *unanticipated* shifts our attention to responses that we could not see coming. Unanticipated responses bring sensations of surprise. Of course, whether you anticipate a response largely depends on your knowledge base, where you live, and who you associate with. So one response that you anticipate, another person may not. To illustrate, read each scenario below. As you read each, think of your mindset at the start of the pandemic and ask yourself whether this is a response you could have anticipated. Why or why not?

- Some governors order roadblocks, forcing cars with out-of-state license plates (especially states with a high infection rate) to turn around or, if they must stay, to self-quarantine.

- People of Asian descent face discrimination and violence from those who blame them for COVID-19.

- Technology companies use robots to ask people if they are experiencing symptoms of COVID-19 and to hand out face masks.

- The number of job postings in public health (e.g., contact tracers), biotechnology, and pharmaceutical fields increases dramatically.

- Some people transform their Little Free Library into a pantry for food, inviting those passing by to take what they need.

- Respiratory droplets emitted from sneezing, coughing, and talking can spread a virus over an entire planet.

Each of these six scenarios could have been anticipated if your social circle included a state trooper, a person of Asian appearance, a robotics engineer, a public health worker, a Little Free Library steward, and a biologist. Certainly, it is impossible to fill your social circle with people from every walk of life, but you can work to expand what you know so that you become skilled at anticipating the unanticipated.

One way is to read widely and take in accounts from a variety of perspectives. Another way is to embrace academic subjects beyond your own that bring a different lens to how you look at the coronavirus pandemic. The payoff of anticipating the unanticipated is that you see more options for how to respond, even in situations where there seem to be few good choices.[5] Just think, reading this short idea paper and taking in the six scenarios above offers a list, albeit incomplete, of how to respond in a pandemic:

- Consider how your travels contribute to the spread of infection. (traveling across state lines)

- Do not scapegoat; know this response is racist and only distracts from finding solutions. (targeting of the Asian population)

- Think outside the box. (robots asking people about symptoms)

- Identify new employment opportunities. (growth in pandemic-related job postings)

- Support vulnerable populations. (Little Free Libraries offering food)

- Realize that small acts—even an uncovered sneeze—can have large effects. (global interconnectedness)

Only when we put in the effort to look beyond our immediate situations and social circles can we see the world in a new light and grasp that things are not what they seem. We must dig deeper and think more broadly to create more possibilities. Then the opportunities and responses we perceive as available to us will be more than they first seemed.

Even sociology as a discipline is more than it seems; it cannot stand alone. Sociology needs biology to study this coronavirus and understand its characteristics that make congregating risky. Sociology needs history to understand how this coronavirus pandemic is different from and similar to past pandemics. Sociology needs math to compare infection and hospitalization rates across populations. Sociology reaches across disciplines to strengthen its capacity to deliver meaningful and relevant analyses, especially in times of crisis.

Joan Ferrante and Chris Caldeira are applied sociologists. They earned their doctorates from the University of Cincinnati and University of California, Davis, respectively. They trust the idea presented in this idea paper because it centers around a sociological concept (anticipated versus unanticipated consequences) that brings no personal agenda to the table. The only way such an agenda can enter is when people refuse, ignore, or cover up what the concept asks them to see. As teachers, they have observed students from different circumstances, cultures, and political orientations apply the concept and come away with new understandings. Ferrante and Caldeira are also part of the Mourning the Creation of Racial Categories Project.

Connect and Reconnect With Food

Sharyn Jones

Anthropology

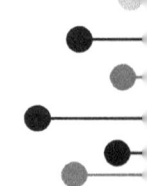

For over 100 years, anthropologists have engaged in the reflective process of asking why their discipline matters. Now, in this time of the COVID-19 crisis, anthropologists, like people in all walks of life, are asking why what we do is important and how it can help us now and in the immediate future.

On a basic level, anthropology is the study of humans. Anthropologists consider what it means to be human, in all its diversity throughout time (past, present, and future) and across the world.[1] For the most part, we all focus on culture. Culture has allowed humans to adapt, survive, and make meaning out of life in every environment throughout human history. By carefully observing people, having conversations with them, and participating in cultures other than our own, anthropologists document the diverse ways people live, behave, think, and believe.

Anthropologists dig deep into the complex systems that humans create to understand and learn from them. But how can this work benefit people in times of crisis? One answer can be found in food. Anthropologists who study this topic direct most of their efforts at understanding the fascinating relationship between humans and what we eat. Some key ideas presented here come from my own research experiences as well as from the generations of anthropologists who have inspired and taught me through their work. The following points provide a foundation:

- Humans connect through food. Eating together is part of being human. To be human is to be part of a community.

- When food systems break down, communities and civilizations collapse.

- Food provides a mode of reconnecting with our humanity, our community, and our Earth, especially in this troubling time.

Humans Connect Through Food

Whether we recognize it or not, humans connect every day with the earth from which their food grows and with those who cook our food and with whom we eat. Of course, we need to eat to live, but we use food in many other ways.[2] If you take the time to reflect on the meaning of food and the needs it serves, it is clear that food brings us comfort, healing, and a way to care for others by nourishing and giving.

The coronavirus pandemic has caused people to think about food in ways they had not before the crisis—the supply chain, shortages, shopping challenges, and storage of surplus foods. People are also thinking more about the less privileged—food insecurity, limited access to affordable and quality food, and risk of infection for supermarket employees. The list could go on.

Consider what you have eaten since the outbreak of COVID-19. No doubt the choices you make about the food you purchase and consume are influenced by your income and occupation. The privileged class—of which I am a member—has adjusted more readily to the stay-at-home and work-from-home mandates. Those of us who have continued to collect an income and work from home likely have the time and resources to engage with food in new, more intimate ways: We are cooking more and using extra time to plan meals and/or share them with family members, partners, and housemates.

This increased engagement with food has given us an opportunity to think about the often-underappreciated connections between food and our health and well-being. It has brought people together in old-timey ways, over the table and through recipes that may reflect a person's heritage or identity. For the first time in many decades, those who live together are now sharing two and even three meals each day. Also, the general public is taking more proactive steps to produce their own food. Online sales of seeds, fruit trees, and live baby chickens, as well as gardening items have increased dramatically.[3] During the pandemic, it is easy to see how we are connected to food and people.

When Food Systems Break Down, Communities and Civilizations Collapse

When someone's income is taken away or reduced, their connection to the food system can break down. The widespread loss of income and other pandemic-induced financial strains exacerbate food and health problems.[4] Those who are less privileged have fewer opportunities to interact with food in the positive ways I describe in the previous section.

The period when unemployment shot up from 3% to 14.4% (30 million unemployed) was a sign of a breakdown in the food system because of compromised income.[5] As a result, poverty and food insecurity drastically increased as more people needed help to feed themselves and their families. A related sign of system breakdown is found in skyrocketing demand for food assistance. Some food banks saw demand increase by 100% to 600%.[6] Drone videos and aerial photos of cars lined up to receive emergency food supplies shocked us. Much of what food banks and pantries distribute comes from supermarket donations, which have cut back on their contributions amid the chaos in the food supply chain, which results in empty shelves.

Health disparities based on race and class have been more starkly defined in the pandemic. Tribal communities in the United States, such as the Navajo Nation, illustrate how food shortages intertwine with poverty and preexisting health conditions to increase a community's susceptibility to COVID-19 infection and hospitalization.[7] Many Navajo peoples struggle with obesity, diabetes, hypertension, substance abuse, high cholesterol, depression, and poor overall health. Food habits are an essential element of most of these diseases. These circumstances are problematic whether or not a person contracts the disease. That is, pandemics impact impoverished communities and countries most acutely. Food plays a key role in these relationships and outcomes.

Likewise, people who cannot work from home, such as those in the food industry (grocery store employees, meat packers, agricultural workers, and many others), put their health and well-being in jeopardy every time they go to work. Their connections with others have also been disrupted because they put their family and friends in more danger if they share space and meals with them.

Food Provides a Mode of Reconnecting With Our Humanity, Our Community, and Our Earth

For people who do not have access to food, there are individuals, groups, and organizations that seek to offer relief, a way of reconnecting them to their humanity. During the COVID-19 crisis, agencies have ramped up programs to address food insecurity in communities with high unemployment, placing special emphasis on children. School employees and bus drivers are delivering food to schoolchildren who would otherwise go without meals. Chefs who can no longer work in restaurants have started cooking and delivering meals to those in need and offering free online cooking workshops. College students are grocery shopping and delivering food to older adults and those who live with them.

The COVID-19 crisis has provided a moment in time when we all can contemplate connecting and reconnecting to people through food. We can think about the past and present role of food in our lives and the future choices about how we intend to use food as a form of connection. Each time we eat, buy food, and share a meal, we can consider the deep and meaningful health implications of what we put into our bodies. We can reflect on what those around us eat and how it affects them. We can think about people who do not have access to healthy food and ask why. We can investigate where the food we buy comes from and examine the entangled food chain that brings each item to the table. We can make efforts to diversify our own meals as well as the food sources that feed us.

When the COVID-19 pandemic has passed, we may have a renewed appreciation for the seemingly simple act of eating. This is an especially important outcome of the crisis because the biggest health concerns for all people are related to nutrition.[8]

Food quality and food security are human dilemmas. There are no simple solutions to the complex issues that humanity faces, such as healthy eating, social inequality, food insecurity, and pandemics. Nevertheless, we can begin to work through these challenges. We can give back and connect with others using food. In this way, I am optimistic that we will move forward with ingenuity, flexibility, and hope.

Sharyn Jones is a professor of anthropology who earned her PhD from the University of Florida. She trusts the ideas presented in this paper because the expanse of human history has illustrated that food is an important part of what makes us human. Humans need community and food provides ways for us to express our appreciation and respect for others. Jones has spent her career studying people and food and has published books, articles, book chapters, and essays on this topic.

3

Look to Science for Answers

Emina Atikovic

Biology

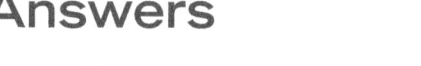
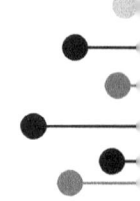

I am a biologist, a scientist who studies life forms—how they came to be (origin and evolution), their physical structure, and how they function and grow. I am, of course, interested in coronaviruses. In 2020, many people learned that *corona*, Latin for "crown," is not just the name of a beer, but rather the name of a family of viruses that has small spikes that extend from their surface.

The coronavirus that causes the disease COVID-19 is the severe acute respiratory syndrome coronavirus 2, or SARS-CoV-2, which belongs to a group of seven known coronaviruses that infects humans.[1] The genetic code of coronaviruses is packaged as RNA.[2] When an RNA virus invades a host cell, it begins making new copies of itself, which then infect other cells in its host. Coronaviruses cause diseases in mammals and birds. In humans, these viruses cause respiratory tract infections from the common cold to the more severe illnesses of SARS, MERS (Middle East respiratory syndrome), and COVID-19 (coronavirus disease, first identified in 2019). Before showing any symptoms of COVID-19, people can be infectious for up to 14 days.

As a scientist, I follow the news in my field. In December of 2019, I read a BBC headline about some mysterious virus that had surfaced in China. My first thought was "Well, that's in a land far, far away from mine." So I went on planning my New Year's celebration. In January of 2020, I saw another article about the same virus. It was spreading.

By March 2020, Bosnia,[3] where I live, was under a complete lockdown. Schools were closed and activities halted. Our restaurants, cafes, malls, movie theaters, shops—all closed—left the entire country in a dormant state. I work at the hospital and live nearby, and, like everyone, I walk to work. One morning, I counted just 10 people on the street (highly unusual because most people walk), all wearing masks and gloves. I got goosebumps! I felt as if I had been thrown into some parallel reality of *The Matrix*, with people trapped in a simulated reality.

I decided to watch *Contagion*. The plot of the film revolves around a fictional RNA virus dubbed MEV-1, inspired by the real-life virus that causes the Nipah virus infection.[4] Nipah has a 40%–75% fatality rate, but the movie presents the virus as having a 25% fatality rate (still very high in comparison to the approximately 2% of COVID-19). In the film, a business executive, played by Gwyneth Paltrow, travels home to Minneapolis from Hong Kong, leaving infectious droplets with every cough, turn of a doorknob, and sexual encounter.

From a biological point of view, the film realistically portrays the vectors by which Nipah spreads from one host to another, although the movie dramatically speeds up the time it takes for the virus to infect a host, for the virus to spread from host to host, and for people to safely develop and mass-produce a vaccine. The film accurately depicts the process by which deadly viruses jump across species (e.g., birds to pigs to humans). This is what screenwriter Scott Z. Burns said about the accuracy of the film: "I didn't want the virus to be divine retribution, or the result of a military conspiracy. I wanted it to be the result of life on Earth in its most mundane. To me, there's something more frightening about what really truly happens in the world."[5,6]

In Bosnia, we lived in isolation and seclusion for two and a half months. It was as if someone had pushed pause, and months later, we were unpaused. When shelter-in-place restrictions were lifted and life went back to its "normal" pace, people started wondering if the restrictions had really been necessary. Conspiracy theories surfaced with unfounded ideas—the virus had been made in a lab; a vaccine is already out there, but "they" do not want to give it to us; and Bill Gates wants to microchip us all.

People started to ask me if COVID-19 is real. Let me just say that the scientific evidence is clear—the coronavirus is real—and the scientific community has verified the identity of the novel coronavirus that causes COVID-19. The questions at this point should not be whether the virus is real or whether it escaped from a lab.[7] The virus is here, and we need to deal with it.

There are more pressing questions: Did we have to put entire countries under complete lockdown to contain it? Was it necessary to throw the global economy into crisis? These questions make sense to ask. Critics argue that if we had not implemented any restrictions, Darwinian natural selection would have happened over time and eventually those people who survived would be immune. However, we would have overwhelmed our health care system and exhausted human resources to care for the sickest. The most vulnerable populations would have suffered and died in the name of "herd immunity" (meaning most of the population is immune). That is the reason Bosnia, and other countries, imposed restrictions on movement and required or recommended masks and gloves. Under lockdown, this minimal social contact lowered the outbreaks of COVID-19 in Bosnia. As a result, we witnessed an extremely low number of people who tested positive, showed symptoms, and died (approximately 3% of those who tested positive).

However, once restrictions were lifted, we saw sharp increases in the number of COVID-19 cases. What does this tell us? That the virus is still "alive." (Technically, the virus is not alive, so it cannot die; rather it gets inactivated.) We must learn to live with it; the virus will not simply disappear.

Biological knowledge allows us to think of how to achieve immunity. Populations can do this in two ways. The first is through herd immunity, in which at least 80% of the population develops an immune response to the virus. Still, scientists do not yet know if people who show immunity, or have produced antibodies, can get sick with COVID-19 a second time.[8] The second way to achieve immunity is to develop a vaccine, which takes time (patience) and money. The challenge for developing a vaccine is isolating the part of the virus that will trigger an immune response without making people sick. At the time of this writing, this is what the world is waiting for.

In the meantime, the best advice is to wash your hands with soap and water frequently. Biology tells us that the coronavirus has a protective shell, a lipid bilayer that is its weakest link. This lipid is a form of fat and therefore can be destroyed by soap and warm water. Those of you who do your dishes by hand know that oily pans are best cleaned with warm water and dish soap. The same concept applies to the coronavirus—the soap deactivates it by dissolving its shell.

If soap and water are not available, then hand sanitizer or disinfectant can be used.[9] These are second choices because they kill just about every microbe on the hands—even the good ones. Be kind to the good microbes; they are our friends and help us to digest food and stave off infections.

When in the presence of other people, always sneeze or cough into your elbow. But if you do, avoid giving elbow high fives. Keep a safe distance from sick people, and do not touch any part of your face until you wash or disinfect your hands. Especially avoid spending prolonged time inside enclosed and windowless (or closed window) environments such as crowded restaurants or office cubicles, which increase the chance of infection.

The amount of time spent with people is an important variable because a person has to be exposed to enough of the virus to become infected. The question is how much is enough. As you might guess, this question is difficult to answer because the amount of virus needed to infect may vary from person to person. One estimate (not verified through experimentation) is 1,000 viral particles.[10] If this is the amount (and that is a big if), then taking just one breath or rubbing an eye can cause infection.[11]

The question of whether a virus is real has been asked during previous pandemics, such as that of HIV and its illness, AIDS. People tend to believe the things they hear repeated, and misinformation about the new coronavirus is no exception. Just because you heard someone say the virus does not exist does not make it true. That is why we must look to science for help in understanding viruses and how to contain them. There are plenty of questions to ask about this coronavirus, but whether it exists is not one of them. That question has been answered.

Emina Atikovic earned her MS degree in biology at the University of Cincinnati. She works as a molecular biologist in a flow cytometry lab at University Clinical Center Tuzla in Bosnia and Herzegovina. She trusts in the process in place to observe and verify that the virus exists. Scientists have isolated this virus, sequenced its genetic code, and proved that it is naturally changing in its genetic structure. The virus that causes COVID-19 is out there, circulating among us.

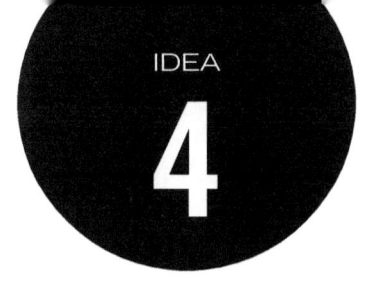

Work to Become Resilient

Isabella Zembrodt

Clinical Counseling

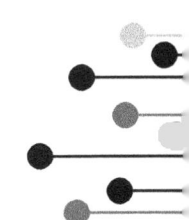

"The world breaks everyone and afterward many are strong at the broken places."

–Ernest Hemingway

Clinical mental health counselors work with clients to address personal challenges and navigate difficult situations. They invite clients to explore new strategies to address entrenched patterns of thinking, behaving, and relating to others. Counselors support clients as they examine how they make decisions, function in relationships, and communicate. The client–therapist relationship plays a central role in the path to problem-solving. The client's trust in the counselor is the foundation of effective intervention aimed at building resilience, the ability to recover from adversity.

Counselors assume that resilience can be learned, and they support clients in this endeavor. One lesson is that adversity is subjective. It is not what happens that determines outcomes; it is how we think about what happens that plays the more important role. Resilient people frame their misfortune in ways that protect them from being overwhelmed. They accurately assess what they can change and then direct their efforts toward it. If we are resilient, we are doing more than surviving; we are finding ways to thrive in the face of adversity. Resilient people become stronger at the broken places.

So what if we try to envision the coronavirus pandemic as an opportunity for building resilience? The COVID-19 crisis disrupted our daily routines, unhinged our sense of control, challenged our beliefs about the world, and threatened our security. It amplified everyday fears, anxieties, stresses, and worries. When unexpected disruptions intrude upon our routines to the point that we reach a state of anxiety and confusion, then we are experiencing trauma. Trauma occurs when some event or encounter violates our expectations and our sense of security. As a result, we may experience emotions such as sadness, anger, and fear, which can give way to hopelessness and helplessness.

Mental health counselors believe that the need to find relief from the effects of trauma can activate resilience. Adverse experiences offer a test of character, an opportunity to clarify priorities, and a chance to identify strengths and draw on them. When we are resilient, we have the capacity to negotiate difficulties and recover from their effects. The work it takes to resolve the effects of trauma can lead to personal growth and positive life changes, including closer relationships, greater confidence, and an enhanced appreciation of life.

Counselors employ multiple counseling interventions, each with specific techniques, to support clients in developing resilience. The name of each therapy hints at the specific technique:

- acceptance and commitment therapy (ACT)

- well-being therapy

- strengths-based therapy

- narrative therapy

- positive psychology

Acceptance and commitment therapy (ACT) emphasizes psychological flexibility, a trait that moves people to adapt to changing circumstances and to address problems in creative ways. The greater the psychological flexibility, the greater the ability to handle painful thoughts and feelings and take effective action. Clients learn to make healthy contact with difficult feelings and thoughts rather than avoid them or feel guilty for having them.

Think about some of the thoughts you have had during the COVID-19 pandemic. You might have a running list of thoughts that do not necessarily connect logically, such as

> I feel afraid to go out and be around people because someone will sneeze on me and I'll get COVID-19. . . . Is this the end of sports? . . . I'm not as invincible as I thought I was even though I'm still young. A couple of friends tested positive and one got really sick and lost twenty pounds. . . . I should move somewhere so I can be closer to nature. . . . I wonder if I'll ever be able to hang out with my friends again without being worried. . . . Should I change careers? . . . I feel so constrained. . . . What if I go out and then bring the virus home to my family? . . . I feel like my world will never be the same. . . . I feel terrible a lot, so I should probably go on medication. . . . If I meet someone, can I date? . . . Sometimes I feel good and think things are going to get better, but then. . . .

Therapists who use the ACT model help clients face difficult thoughts, feelings, and memories and work with them to accept and embrace them with an eye toward taking effective action. Therapists also point out that some of these thoughts are fleeting and will change. In other words, we do not need to be imprisoned by every thought we have.

Another type of resilience-building therapy is *well-being therapy*. Mental health is more than the absence of disease; it is a state of well-being. And well-being is more than surviving; it is thriving. Clients develop well-being when they accept reality, identify their strengths, and commit to taking actions that will help them achieve satisfaction within their lives, work, relationships, and accomplishments. Clients thrive when they can use adversity as a catalyst to make life better for their families and communities. As a result, they develop a sense of purpose, life satisfaction, and well-being. The following passage describes using well-being therapy for the development of a solution in response to adversity.

A licensed massage therapist is devastated because their practice has collapsed as a result of COVID-19. They are on unemployment and have not worked since their state went into lockdown. Their clients are mostly adults of older age and people with underlying health conditions who benefit from massage. Massage is classified as "extremely high risk" for spreading the virus, as it is impossible to stand six feet from a client to avoid prolonged exposure. And massage therapy is classified as a "nonessential service" even though it is essential to many in pain and discomfort. In addition, massage therapists cannot easily acquire N95 masks, which are made available to essential medical workers only. Even if the massage therapist were able to return to work, liability insurance will not cover any claims related to COVID-19 transmission. While it is hard to accept these circumstances as the reality, they must. What is the massage therapist to do? They decide to find a new career in which their massage therapy skills and knowledge can be used. They identify two possibilities: study to be a veterinary assistant/technician to help pets that suffer from conditions that can be eased through massage therapy, or study to be a physical therapist in which their knowledge of anatomy would be an advantage.

Strengths-based therapy engages clients in discussions about their strengths—their skills, talents, areas of knowledge, and social connections. Counselors encourage clients to look at their daily life for evidence of their strengths. First, clients think about what life would be like if they were to quit doing what they do regularly. For example, how would life be for themselves and others if the coronavirus outbreak led them to stop paying their bills, cleaning up after themselves, or helping their neighbors? The answers point to a person's strengths: reliability, conscientiousness, cleanliness, and compassion. Second, counselors ask clients to monitor how they handle the adversity as it unfolds, reminding them to try not to be overwhelmed and to focus only on taking the next best action.

We cannot know how things will turn out, but we can try to focus on the positive and stay present. Being open to new ways of thinking and doing without fixating on all that is going wrong and could go wrong is one way to move forward. We cannot know what will happen—or what we are capable of—until we put our strengths to the test. Strong people "know how to organize their suffering so as to bear only the most necessary pain."[1]

In *narrative therapy*, counselors ask clients to tell their story. The psychologist Viktor Frankl reminds us that people can withstand the most difficult hardships when they can make sense of their stories.[2] Traumas leave traces that alter the brain in ways that damage how people interpret and respond. Counselors use narrative therapy to revise memories by framing the adverse event in a larger context, encouraging clients to make room for new stories and interpretations. That is, clients benefit from seeing that there is more to the story or that other factors were shaping the actions. Changing someone's narrative can transform them from victim to survivor.

Narrative therapy helps a client understand how the way they tell the story of their lives affects the way they think and behave. If the story is not helpful, the therapist helps the client tell the story in a way that is empowering. The goal is to construct a story that gives the client a positive identity. This process takes place over multiple sessions in which clients tell their story, analyze it for truth, and rewrite it in a meaningful way. Narrative therapy prompts clients to ask what life wants from them at this time and how they can transcend their situation and transform their story. Can they envision ways to find happiness? The lesson here is that we can be the authors of our own life stories.

Counselors encourage clients to revise and create new narratives with compassion and an emphasis on their strengths and lessons learned. For example, during a therapy session, a client mentions that his loss of employment due to COVID-19 has led him to receive food from the local food bank. The client talks of being in a food line for the first time in his life and not feeling comfortable. He speaks about feeling ashamed for not being able to provide for his children. Through discussion with the therapist, the client works out a new narrative that reframes his story of relying on the food bank: "You lost your job through no fault of your own. Obviously, you care about being a good parent to your children. There is nothing wrong with asking for help. Try to see that you are supporting your family and that this is an act of strength. Accept this food as a gift that volunteers are offering during a difficult time."

Narrative therapy helps revise the story by changing the meaning of what happened. Instead of interpreting the loss of a job as a failure, a person can see it as an opportunity to open and rethink how to live life. Their new narrative could recognize that they are not alone in losing their job. By rewriting the story about standing in a food line, the actions become about supporting family, accepting gifts, and relying on others.

Positive psychology builds resilience by focusing on the experiences that make life worth living. It puts the emphasis on happiness, the key elements of which are positive emotion, engagement, and purpose. Positive emotions counter negativity. Such emotions come from purposefully engaging in experiences and making efforts to feel joy, gratitude, hope, pride, awe, and love. We know we are engaged when we are absorbed in positive activities and interactions and are not resorting to self-absorption. When we have purpose, life is meaningful because we are in the service of something bigger than the self.

During this crisis, I have learned of many clients engaging in positive acts to bring relief to others and to reassure them that they matter. One client delivers lunches to schoolchildren who have no food at home. Another writes thank you messages on their sidewalks and driveways for mail carriers and delivery drivers. I have seen clients become more present in their family life and find creative ways to celebrate special moments, including drive-by graduations, birthday parties, memorial services, and window visits where loved ones "touch" hands against the window.

The pandemic has taught us that we do not live in isolation. We are interdependent. We cannot win when some lose. It has forced us to change how we interact. How we manage and adapt to this unexpected change determines how we come out of it.

Isabella Zembrodt is a licensed professional clinical counselor (LPCC). She earned her doctorate of educational leadership at Northern Kentucky University. She trusts the idea that resilience can be learned because she frequently observes people discovering their strengths and using them to overcome adversity and create a better life for themselves, their families, and their communities. Her latest research is about identifying factors that predict educational persistence among low-income college students.

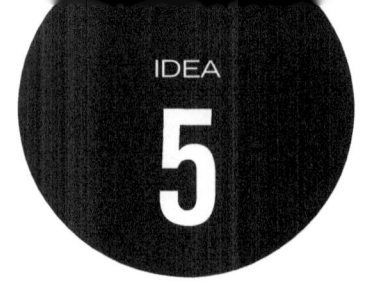

IDEA

5

Engage in New Ways

Mark Neikirk

Community Engagement

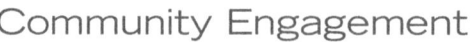
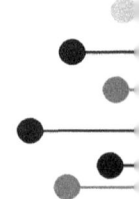

In the context of higher education, community engagement connects students to the community, with benefits for both. Such connections enhance student learning while also addressing community needs.[1] A psychology class might design, disseminate, and analyze a survey for a local nonprofit seeking to improve a service. An art class might produce murals for a city streetscape. A social work class might mentor youth at a community center.

Lockdowns and social distancing strained the ability of higher education to do community engagement—but not to the breaking point. Long before the new coronavirus appeared, colleges and universities were already integrating community engagement into online courses, creating more flexibility in designing and carrying out engagement.[2] Social distancing did not launch online community engagement experiences; it only accelerated them.

In this idea paper, I explore the benefits of the flexibility that online engagement offers in times of crisis, using examples from the Mayerson Student Philanthropy Project at Northern Kentucky University. Our student philanthropy model looks like this:

- Each class receives $2,000 to invest.

- The classes identify community needs, each using the lens of its particular discipline.

- Students search for nonprofit organizations that address those needs and invite them to write a request for funding.

- After evaluating what they have learned about each request, students decide which projects to fund.

For example, a sports marketing class might identify a need, such as combating ALS, breast cancer, or food insecurity. Because the class is focused on sports and marketing, students would seek nonprofits that are in some way involved in sports. Perhaps the agency plans to host a 10K run, a golf tournament, or a bowl-a-thon to build awareness and raise funds. Students next invite such organizations to write a request for funding outlining how they might use $2,000 to offset the expenses related to marketing their event. The students review the submitted proposals, visit any agencies they want to consider further, and, ultimately, choose an agency as their recipient. They might also volunteer to help with the agency's marketing effort.

When COVID-19 hit, the rapid conversion to complete online instruction was a stress test for universities that wanted to keep their campuses and communities connected and to maintain the demonstrable benefits of community engagement. A computer science class and a law class on our campus serve as two cases in point.

In the first case, a computer science class had been divided into several teams, with each team assigned to work with a nonprofit client to deliver a tailored IT solution, such as a website improvement, a data reporting protocol, or an inventory tracking system. Each participating nonprofit received an IT solution customized to its needs, and one was to be selected by the class to receive $2,000 toward the cost of putting the solution in place.[3]

When the coronavirus forced the students to leave their classrooms and the staffs of the nonprofits to transition to working from home, communication between the student teams and their chosen nonprofits suffered as new, unanticipated urgencies took precedence for both parties. However, one of the student teams pressed forward, switching from in-person communication to an online platform using voice, video, and text to communicate. It was that team's nonprofit partner that received the $2,000 from the class as a whole.

Consider the client-management lessons gained by these future computer scientists. They learned the importance of keeping the lines of communication open, no matter the extenuating circumstances. Community engagement values real-world navigation. Is there anything more probable in the real world than extenuating circumstances?

In the second class, law students worked on legal cases representing children and families. Their cases typically involve custody complications, child abuse, immigration issues, or other hardships. For the philanthropy component, the students looked at community agencies focused on children and families caught in such circumstances. After COVID-19 emerged, the students reexamined those agencies to understand their needs in the pandemic. The students were anxious to invest in helping the agencies adapt to COVID-19 exigencies. As one student in the class explained, "This opened a whole new side of many of these organizations as they scrambled to adjust to the pandemic."

The class awarded a grant to the Women's Crisis Center, a domestic abuse shelter that traditionally houses clients and their children together at group homes. The highly contagious nature of the virus made a group living situation impractical, so the center placed its clients in individual rooms at local hotels. The law students awarded funds to assist with that expense.

As with the computer science class, the law class was introduced to the real world's propensity to shuffle the deck. Students in both classes were challenged to play the hand they were dealt, which they were able to do, to the benefit of their partnering agencies. These two examples show how community engagement can adapt to changing circumstances and also remain productive. Students used web searches, Zoom, and other virtual tools to identify funding opportunities. And the reflective essay, an essential component of community engagement classes, was easily adaptable to the virtual environment, through blog posts, video uploads, or Zoom dialogues.

The process may change, but the principles of community engagement hold. Students must always value listening to the community and tailor their engagement work accordingly. The COVID-19 crisis presented an opportunity for adaptation and creativity. In such a cataclysmic environment, the call to action is to rethink—not stop.

Not stopping—pressing forward as circumstances mutate—forces students to ask, "What now?" If they were in sports marketing class and sports activities halt, is that the end? No, not if the students and the community agencies trust each other to be creative and adapt. Suppose a 10K run was planned on city streets with thousands starting and finishing together. That cannot happen in a pandemic. Might it be reinvented as a 10K that you run alone or with your dog in your neighborhood, uploading snapshots to a common website or social media? The question, then, becomes how students can support the revised model.

Students can find new ways to engage with nonprofit organizations and the communities they serve. We can reasonably expect the shift to online communication to outlast the pandemic. And the reasons why community engagement came to be in the first place—connecting the campus and the community to benefit both—will remain through the crisis, which makes community engagement even more necessary.

The point is, disruptive circumstances need not end a planned project. Rather, the disruption is best seen as an opportunity to energize the class. That is particularly true for a class with a philanthropy component. After all, philanthropy is always called upon in times of disruption. It's after a hurricane that relief efforts are most needed, after a factory closes that the workers need job training, or after a pandemic shuts down group homes that a women's shelter needs hotel rooms for its clients.

Mark Neikirk is the executive director of the Scripps Howard Center for Civic Engagement, which connects classrooms with community partners and projects. The center is the home of the Mayerson Student Philanthropy Project. Twelve years of observation and data gathering reveal that students and faculty can take the basic model for student philanthropy and invigorate it with their own ideas to benefit the classroom and community. Neikirk is the former managing editor of The Cincinnati Post, *where he was committed to giving the community a voice in each day's newspaper.*

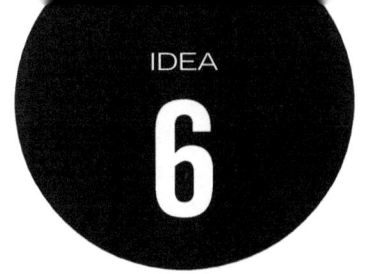

Slow Down, Pause, Reflect

Kelly Moffett

Creative Writing

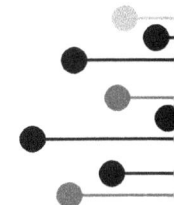

The field of creative writing is grounded in the imagination and the human capacity for inventiveness. Three main genres of creative writing are taught at the college level: fiction, creative nonfiction, and poetry. I focus primarily on poetry. It is what I write, read, teach, and long for—especially in times of crisis.[1]

Poet and critic Edward Hirsch writes, "I am convinced the kind of experience . . . one gets from poetry cannot be duplicated elsewhere."[2] The kind of experience I concentrate on here is a contemplative process. It is a conscious act of slowing down when our minds are rushing forward in a haze of anxiety, confusion, and overinformation. It involves a sudden attentiveness.

During the COVID-19 crisis, I received an email from a student saying, "I have been writing ghazals in quarantine. It has been helping me quite a bit!" A ghazal is a form of poetry that expresses loss and pain, written in rhyming couplets. I love that this student is finding poetry helpful. But why does poetry help? Because the student is experiencing the benefits of an engaged contemplative practice.

One way to describe what poetry can do for the mind is to compare the experience of poetry to the heightened awareness that comes when traveling to a country where everyday routines feel different and things look unfamiliar. When we do not know the language, we pay more attention, pausing to take in the freshness of the adventure, bit by bit.

In February of 2020, I traveled to a university in Romania to teach a creative writing course. We were still in the early stages of the pandemic, before mandated social distancing. As soon as I arrived, even though exhausted from the jet lag of the seven-hour difference, I felt compelled to explore.

I challenged myself not to take pictures with my phone. I decided that if I saw something worthy of memory, I would stop, gaze, and create a simile of what I saw to really take in what I was seeing. For example, on my first night, while walking through the old part of town on a medieval cobbled street, I looked up at the lights strung above my head. They were drawn across the narrow street at a height of about fifteen feet—so beautiful against the night sky it was almost painful.

Instead of taking a photo, I asked myself, what does each lightbulb look like? How could I describe this to others? And then it came to me: like a raindrop frozen above me, like a tulip about to flower. While I could not find the precise comparison that would bring this moment to life for those back home, what was important was that this exercise replicated precisely what happens when we read or write a poem. My heightened awareness made me pause and concentrate only on the lights and how I might describe them.

The self-isolation resulting from the COVID-19 outbreak has forced us all to slow down physically, but with this crisis at our doorsteps, our minds are like beehives, a frenetic energy feeding off of anxiety. When the Queen of England addressed her nation, she expressed hope that self-isolation may "present an opportunity to slow down, pause, and reflect in prayer or meditation."[3] When in the center of a crisis, I am not sure if I am ready for reflection. But my mind, my whole body, longs to slow down, pause, reflect.

Back at home each day, my dog and I walk to a pond to watch a family of turtles sunning. There are at least five babies and two others large enough to be parents and another far larger—I like to think of him as the grandpa—that has a thick layer of green algae on his shell. He likes to let all four limbs hang as he balances on the very tip of a log. Just stopping to truly see this turtle family helps me pause. I look, pay attention, and almost narrate to myself what I am seeing to be sure I am fully present, fully focused.

I also like to pause at a lip of the pond, take off my sunglasses, and look into the water. It is funny how I have to tell myself to look, to register exactly what I perceive, and eventually I see forms under the water: the fish body, the turtle silhouette. And sometimes I like to see what mood the pond is in. If it is taking in the images of the clouds above, still and quiet, a reflection only, or if it ripples and obscures what is under the surface. Ripples—such a sensuous word, a word that sounds like its meaning.

These experiences show what it is like to be mindful. But how to be mindful with language? We take language for granted as we talk, listen, and read. We become overwhelmed at all the language coming at us, often without paying attention to the words. Poetry makes us pay attention, word by word. I liken it to laying bricks. Whether composing or reading poetry, we have to hold each word as a brick, feel the weight of it, understand its texture, and place it securely, checking to see that it is placed properly before reaching for the next brick. In other words, we are forced to slow down, to go word by word/brick by brick and become fully attentive in the process.

I suggest to beginning poetry students that they read, and really take in the words, of at least one poem per day. Here is an excerpt from a poem by celebrated Swedish poet Tomas Tranströmer that I read early in the quarantine period.

> *A man feels the world with his work like a glove.*
> *He rests for a while at midday having laid aside the gloves on a shelf.*
> *There they suddenly grow, spread*
> *and black out the whole house from inside.*

A man feels the world with his work like a glove.

The first line forces me to pause. What does it mean for a man to feel the world like a glove? I am not sure. But I stop. And I think, "No, it is not that he feels the world like a glove; he feels the world with his work." This is not the kind of language that I encounter in conversation or in emails or in the news. I do not know exactly what it means, but I linger. Then linger some more. And I am not frustrated. I am enthralled. My mind, even without me realizing it, has stopped. Then I am given more delightful language.

He rests for a while at midday having laid aside the gloves on a shelf.

I see them there. Dark shadows on a white shelf.

There they suddenly grow, spread and black out the whole house from inside.

In my mind, I am there. The gloves have grown. They have taken up the whole space of the house. I see them looking out a window. What does this line mean? I could guess, but I do not want to. I want to stay in the image. Rest in that final line. It feels so good to stop my mind from the whir of anxiety. Like a long and deep stretch. I did not even realize until reading that poem how quickly my mind was moving.

French philosopher Simone Weil believed that "absolutely unmixed attention is prayer."[4] And French philosopher Nicolas Malebranche wrote the maxim "Attentiveness is the natural prayer of the soul."[5] If I could rewrite the quote, it would be "Poetry is the natural prayer of the soul." The definitions of prayer are immense, but I like to think of it as being *present* to a *presence* of language and life, all of the beautiful, small things, such as an image of a glove on a shelf, or a turtle family.

For this reason, I love this segment of the poem "A Green Stream" by Chinese poet Wang Wei.[6] The poet is simply present to the presence of nature around him.

Rapids hum on scattered stones,
Light is dim in the close pines,
The surface of an inlet sways with nut-horns,
Weeds are lush along the banks.
Down in my heart, I have always been clear
As this clarity of waters.

Wang Wei takes in the stones, the pines, the nut-horns, the weeds, and in so doing, finds that his true self "Down in my heart" is as clear as the stream's water. We only have to allow ourselves to be present.

Writing and reading poetry can also be considered contemplative practices—processes that facilitate a state of calm centeredness, which supports expression and insight. Consider having your own contemplative practice. Start by looking up a poem a day at websites such as Poetry Daily or Verse Daily. I hope that each poem inspires you to be ever more attentive to the world that presents itself to you. And perhaps this attentiveness will inspire you to write. I hope that it does. You, too, can build something word by word (brick by brick) and feel the delicious sensation of a mind that has slowed down, calmed, and stilled like a pond on a sunny afternoon in spring.

Kelly Moffett teaches poetry and creative writing and earned her MFA at West Virginia University. She often retreats to Trappist monasteries to study silence and engage in contemplative creativity. She trusts that slowing down, pausing, and reflection are contemplative practices that support reading and writing poetry, because both require complete presence to focus on the task at hand. The health benefits include strengthened immune functioning, decreased stress levels, and better performance. Moffett is the author of one chapbook and three poetry collections, with a fourth coming out soon. Her poetry has been published in many journals, and one of her poems is in the Verse Daily archives. In 2019, she taught creative writing as a Fulbright Scholar at Universitatea Babeş-Bolyai in Romania. Her stay was cut short by the COVID-19 pandemic.

Grasp the Deeper Meaning of Social Distancing

Joan Ferrante and Prince Brown Jr.
with poetry and screenwriting by India Hackle

Critical White Studies

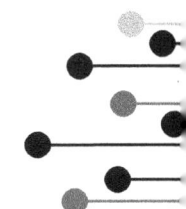

Critical white studies is a transdisciplinary field that addresses, among other things, how *White* became a label for a racial category.[1] Specifically, it considers how diverse peoples came to identify only as White. This field of study brings awareness to the laws and social practices that qualified some for membership into the White category while excluding others. It examines the histories and effects of white privilege, dominance, and supremacy. Scholars also look at peoples within the White category who self-identify and/or are denigrated as "white trash."

One basic tenet of critical white studies is that the White category distinguished itself from other racial categories by physically distancing itself from those it deemed non-white. *Physical distancing* calls to mind the *social distancing* that has defined the COVID-19 pandemic. In this context, the distancing refers to the actions people have taken to limit gatherings and put at least six feet of physical space between themselves and others, with the aim of reducing the spread of COVID-19.

Mandating physical space between people is not a new practice in the United States. For over 400 years, governments at all levels created ordinances and laws evicting and barring non-white-classified[2] peoples from spaces the White-classified claimed as their own. The White category treated the non-white classified peoples, but especially the Black-classified, as dangerous—as if they could infect white spaces. Physical distancing allowed those in the White category to control and monopolize valued resources—the best land, housing, and jobs.

Legally mandated physical distancing was dismantled when the military was ordered to integrate (1948), educational segregation was declared unconstitutional (1954), Jim Crow laws were disbanded (1965), and discrimination in renting and selling homes was declared illegal (1968). However, making physical distancing illegal has not ended segregation and discrimination or provided disenfranchised people with the resources to enroll in better quality schools, move to better housing, and access experiences that cost money.

This history of physical distancing helps explain the segregation that exists still today. We know that the past has reached into the present because we all can think of ways we feel, and actually are, separated from people in other racial categories. For you, it might be apparent when you picture your neighborhood, church, residence hall cafeteria, or when you experience a "strained smile in a grocery store."[3]

The devastating effects of such separations are evident when we examine COVID-19's infection and death rates by racial category. Where people live, learn, work, and play affects the chances of becoming infected, being hospitalized, and surviving COVID-19. Racial and ethnic minorities are more likely to live in neighborhoods without nearby grocery stores, making it more difficult to shelter in place. They are more likely to live in homes with limited space and more people, as often occurs in multigenerational households. And overrepresentation in jails, prisons, and detention centers brings increased risk that comes with congregate living.

In the space of this paper, we cannot explore all the resulting disparities of extreme distancing measures that the White category has instituted over hundreds of years. Here we will focus on the ways that the White-classified have physically distanced from the Native American and Black categories, but know that the White category has physically distanced itself from the Asian, Hispanic,[4] and Hawaiian-Pacific Islander[5] categories as well. We draw on a poem and a scene from a screenplay to emotionally engage with lived experiences.

The Indian-Classified

When we review statistics on coronavirus infections and deaths, data for the Native American category are rarely listed. Among the states that do report data, we see disproportionate suffering. For example, in Arizona, Native Americans are just 6% of the population but account for 16% of the state's COVID-19 deaths. In New Mexico, the Native American category makes up less than 10% of the population, but it accounts for 45% of known cases.[6,7] News headlines illustrate these imbalances:

- Native Americans left out of U.S. coronavirus data and labelled as "other"[8]

- Navajo Nation reels under weight of the coronavirus—and history of broken promises[9]

- Doctors Without Borders arrives in New Mexico to help Native Americans battle the coronavirus[10]

The roots of the racial disparities, made even more apparent during the COVID-19 crisis, can be traced to the long history of physical distancing. Specifically, since the founding of Jamestown in 1607, governments have enacted laws removing 2,000 distinct indigenous societies from their lands. Those laws forced Indian-classified populations to move or be removed.

All the lands we now call the United States were gradually and violently broken into pieces to be discovered, claimed, fought over, fenced in, sold, and purchased by those almost exclusively in the White category. In the end, Indian-classified peoples owned less than 2% of the land they once controlled and managed.[11] In addition, Indian-classified children were removed from their families and cultures to be adopted into White-classified families and communities. Adoption and land removal were part of the national policy known as "Kill the Indian, Save the Man." That policy held that the Indian-classified could become White if they were extracted from their communities and subjected to socialization into the ways of the dominant group.

The poem "My Dear" by India Hackle offers a glimpse of the past. It draws on the words from two letters Andrew Jackson wrote to his wife in 1813, when he was leading a battle against the Creek Nation.[12]

My Dear,

[We] have mounted men to destroy the Creek Town Talus, [we] executed in elegant stile. [We] behaved like what I expected— behaved bravely and as I could wish.
Leaving dead on the field   one hundred & seventy-six,
taking prisoners   eighty. Among these an infant boy,
suckling the lifeless breast of his Indian mother.
[I] asked the Captive women to care for the child—they refused.
They said, "All his relations are dead, kill him too!"
Their words thrilled through. I took the infant in my own tent— with my own hands fed him sugared water.

I send [this] little Indian boy,
take care of him—for all his family is destroyed—
Keep [him] in the house. He is a Savage
[but one] that fortune has thrown in my hands
I therefore want him well taken care of,
he may have been given to me for some Valuable purpose—
in fact, when I reflect that he is so much like myself
I feel an unusual "sympathy" for him—
tell my dear little Andrew to treat him well—

In haste, your affectionate Husband

In this letter, the interpersonal dynamics that made physical distancing a reality are described in the words of the remover. This war removed 256 Indian-classified people through death or imprisonment. It was one event of many that cleared the land to become the states of Alabama and Georgia. Amid the devastation, a baby was violently extracted from his family and community and adopted into the Jackson family. The "savage" child, pulled from the hands of Creek women planning to mercifully kill him, was sent to live with Jackson's wife and son under the command to care for him and treat him well.

The Black-Classified

The COVID-19 statistics on infections, hospitalizations, and deaths for the Black-classified are startling. In Michigan, the Black-classified comprise 14% of the population but constitute 40% of deaths. In St. Louis, they are 45% of the population and 64% of all COVID-19 cases. And in New York City, death rates among Black-classified persons (92.3 deaths per 100,000) are double those of the White-classified (45.2 per 100,000).[13]

While many practices against Black-classified people have manifested in such disparities, here we will focus on Jim Crow, a system of legal segregation barring the Black-classified from spaces claimed by the White-classified.[14] In the words of Malcolm X, the Jim Crow laws shouted at the Black-classified, "You can't live here, you can't enter here, you can't eat here, drink here, walk here, work here, you can't ride here, you can't play here, you can't study here."[15]

The punishments for violating Jim Crow laws varied, including fines, imprisonment, and violence. But the ultimate punishment was lynching. Lynching is a premeditated and terrorist action in which White-identifying people appoint themselves to be the judge, jury, and executioner of the person they have defined as a transgressor into their spaces. Often, mobs watched, urging executioners on, taking pictures, and removing pieces of the lynched victim's clothing as souvenirs. These actions are described in excerpted scenes from India Hackle's screenplay based on the book *Time of Terror* by James Cameron, a firsthand account of his surviving an attempted lynching. The scene begins after the mob has just lynched two of Cameron's friends and then turn to Cameron. An unidentified person in the crowd screams for them to stop, and for an inexplicable reason, the mob does.

Lynching Tree. Night.

SMALL VOICE

Let him go now. He didn't have nothing to do with it.
He's one of the good ones.

The MOB *quiets, then is silent. The* THREE WHITE MEN *tying the noose around the neck of* JAMES *show expressions of embarrassment and slowly take it off, then lead him down the path, back to the jailhouse. The* MOB *is silent and wears expressions of shame and embarrassment. When* JAMES *moves off camera the* MOB *begins to dwindle and when completely gone, A pickup truck drives up and parks close to the tree where the* TWO BLACK HANGING BODIES *are.* A YOUNG WHITE MAN *gets out the pickup truck and uses a small knife to cut off small pieces of clothing from the hanging bodies. He exits.*

Voice-Over of WHITE CELLMATE to JAMES

I'm sorry this is where we are. That this is who we are. You know my son was out there, too? He could have been the one that tied the rope around your neck.

A WHITE FATHER *with his* LITTLE WHITE GIRL *walk toward the* TWO BLACK HANGING BODIES. *The* LITTLE WHITE GIRL *(excitedly) points to one hanging body. The* WHITE FATHER *reaches up and cuts a piece of hair off that body. They exit.*

Voice-Over of WHITE CELLMATE to JAMES

I didn't teach nothing like this to him. Seem like it came out the soil and crawled up in him, but he didn't try and shake it off. He just let it catch 'round his leg, his man, his heart. I told him it wasn't right— to watch people get killed like that. That something was off about him now. That something had fallen off . . .

We watch as a WHITE MALE TEENAGER *and* WHITE FEMALE TEENAGER *come into view and take the shoes off the feet of the* TWO BLACK HANGING BODIES. *They exit.*

The lynching scene highlights the spectrum of ways the White-classified participated in this extreme act of physical distancing. There are the executioners, the mob, the souvenir-takers, and an excited child absorbing the "lessons." The audacity of these acts requires all involved to feel superior (or learn to act that they feel superior) over bodies they perceive as unequal. It requires that they feel certain the act was deserved. The Black-classified are not terrorized only by the men and women who tie the rope and take souvenirs but by the lack of voices yelling stop and observers moving to take action. They are terrorized by cellmates and those who protest with empty words: "I did not teach this; I am not racist, I have no explanation."

At the time of this writing, Ahmaud Arbery—a Black-classified man—was fatally shot by two White-identifying men who claimed to be making a citizen's arrest. They hunted down the jogging Arbery, cornered him, and took his life. Another Black-classified man, George Floyd, was killed by a White-identifying officer who pinned his knee on Floyd's neck for almost nine minutes. (Note that we use the word White-identifying here because such acts suggest the perpetrator is heavily invested in their whiteness.)

Many White-classified people quietly know and fear that their neighborhood is not welcoming to their Black-classified friends. When extreme acts of physical distancing such as a citizen's arrest and police brutality unfold daily, reflect on your response. Do you meet these acts with confusion about how they could possibly occur? Do you wonder how can they be quickly resolved? Or do you think that perhaps the victims "deserved" it?

The White-identifying and White-classified may feel the impulse to distance themselves from both the past and present by thinking, "I would never do this! It is not relevant to me." But the call to action begins with this question: "Are there concrete examples in my life story that tell me I would respond in a way that is different from the spectrum of responses described in this idea paper?"

The acts of physical distancing, past and present, covered in this paper are not isolated—each is part of a chain of events hundreds of years long. And while we might like to think the events of the past do not reach into the present, their legacy is exposed and laid bare by the disproportionate manner in which the COVID-19 virus impacts communities of color.

These dramatic differences did not just come "out the soil and crawl up" on us. If we take a long view that encompasses past to present, the answer is that Indian-classified tribes were removed. The answer is that the Black-classified were barred from entering spaces or that White-identifying mobs ran them out at some point. For 400 years, the message has been clear: Get out of our spaces or who knows what will happen to you.

Joan Ferrante is a professor of sociology, and Prince Brown Jr. is an emeritus professor of sociology. Ferrante earned her PhD from the University of Cincinnati, and Brown from Boston University. They are the editors of The Social Construction of Race and Ethnicity in the United States. *India Hackle is a graduate student in the creative writing program at Cornell University. All three are part of the* Mourning the Creation of Racial Categories Project, *as director, consultant, and artistic co-director, respectively. They trust what they write about physical distancing because the laws and policies mandating it can be readily found. Eyewitness accounts in letters and autobiographies add further evidence.*

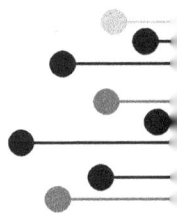

Change the Story, Change What Is Possible

John Alberti

Cultural Studies

The field of cultural studies seeks to understand cultural processes in the context of a capitalist-driven global economy. It explores power dynamics, social relations, and individual experiences in contemporary culture.[1] To do this, the discipline draws on many other disciplines, such as anthropology, English, sociology, and communications. Cultural studies puts the focus on the ways people give expression to their values and beliefs.

Take, for example, the U.S. national anthem. Hearing the anthem is a ritual familiar to most of us but no less remarkable for that familiarity. Before a sporting match begins, for instance, we listen to the national anthem. For most of us, it is almost impossible to hear without having an emotional reaction. Some find themselves misting up, others feel a growing irritation. Yet neutrality is rarely an option; in some powerful way, the song defines our identity.

We can think of national anthems as miniature, poetic, musical stories about the nations they represent and the citizens who live there.[2] These national anthems affect us powerfully. Even people who do not really know the words (or what "ramparts" means) can still feel a powerful emotional pull (or push) when they hear them. An anthem impacts us because it is a story.

A national anthem illustrates a key idea in cultural studies: Stories matter. Stories are how we make sense of what is happening in the world and in our daily lives. By "making sense," I mean creating a perspective of order and predictability, of assigning purpose and meaning to that which can seem random and chaotic. When we refer to "the coronavirus pandemic," for example, we are invoking the *story* of the coronavirus, implying that eventually there will be a beginning, a middle, and an end, that there will be heroes and villains, and ultimately, a kind of moral to that story.

We can readily see that there are already multiple stories contending for the role of what is real in the story of the current pandemic. What was once a hoax, for example, became a war against the virus, or a war over wearing masks. The words "hoax" and "war" evoke two kinds of story lines, each with a different set of expectations and feelings. These stories do not simply coexist but compete with each other for popularity and influence.

This concept points to another key idea of cultural studies: Stories are always interwoven with social and political power, and not just stories that are obviously political. Songs (such as national anthems), sayings, memes, and even jokes are types of stories that gain popularity through what they suggest about how power works. If stories express how we believe power works, then they also express how we believe the world operates.

Cultural studies teaches us that stories are always unstable by nature and that official stories, in particular, need constant renewal and reinforcement to stay relevant. Even the simplest of stories can be interpreted in multiple ways, and the lived experiences of those who read or hear stories dramatically affect how they understand them, and not always in predictable ways.

The concept of hegemony, or how one social group maintains dominance over others, helps us think critically about how stories matter. We know that dominance can result from physical force, but the concept of hegemony also helps us understand how stories can reinforce that dominance, can convince people of the rightness of the way things are. We call the stories that support the status quo *dominant stories*.

The idea of *dominant stories* does not refer only to the pronouncements of government officials or to the recognized narratives taught in history classes. Dominant stories also include "common sense" beliefs, like the idea that if you work hard and believe in yourself, you can overcome any obstacle. Think of the popularity of "rags to riches" stories, for example, tales of how someone begins with nothing and rises to a position of power, fame, and influence, all through personal determination.[3]

These dominant stories create an overall attitude and acceptance of certain core values and beliefs. However, they are neither all-encompassing nor all-powerful. Dominant stories are still just that—stories—and like all stories, they contain complex meanings that can be read in contradictory ways, especially when two dominant values—say, self-sacrifice and ambition—come into conflict.

Still other kinds of stories—residual and emergent stories—can counter hegemonic dominant stories.[4] *Residual stories* refer to cultural narratives that continue to have emotional power and a strong sense of purpose long after the historical age that produced them has passed. Religious stories, folk stories, and even fairy tales fall into this category, as can historical artworks. These cultural narratives stay alive because they are reimagined and repurposed to shed a light on our lives as they are lived today. They can also be used to deliberately counter dominant stories. As a case in point, over four centuries ago, Shakespeare's *Macbeth* was thought to have been first performed by an all-male cast. In 2020, Misfits Theater Company repurposed the play into an all-female and nonbinary production. Macbeth is presented as a woman warrior with a wife, Lady Macbeth.[5] In this sense, the residual story of *Macbeth* stays relevant at the same time that it challenges the dominant gender-binary construct.

Emergent stories also counter dominant stories, arising out of their contradictions and often turning them back on themselves.[6] We can think of emergent stories as protest stories, and they have played a long and important role in American history, from the abolition of slavery to the granting of voting rights for women. These stories craft new futures that the dominant stories dismissed as impossible, impractical, and contrary to the "natural order."

Abolitionist movements of the 19th century, for example, used the "all men are created equal" story line in the Declaration of Independence to tell a different story of America, one built on hypocrisy. One such story is "What to the Slave is the Fourth of July?," a speech by Frederick Douglass, who demanded that the nation live up to its purported values of equality and democracy. His fiery, satirical rhetoric worked to connect head and heart. He knew that the future is a story, and that in order to work for a better future, we need to imagine it. Central to that work is abandoning—or revising—old narratives, and creating new and better ones.

But what does this all mean for us right now, in the middle of the COVID-19 pandemic? It means that this crisis creates new openings and new opportunities for other stories, for residual and emergent stories, to come to the fore. We have already seen how several emergent stories have moved out of the margins to the political mainstream. For example, the idea of a universal basic income is a story teaching us that "the more we are apart, the more we realize how much we need each other." It counters the "pull yourself up by the bootstraps" story. Former presidential candidate Andrew Yang's call to give all American adults $1,000 per month, labeled as a "fringe" idea by previous politicians, became a central part of the Coronavirus Aid, Relief, and Economic Security Act (CARES Act), which addresses the economic fallout of stay-at-home orders.

Even more dramatically, the idea, movement, and emergent story of Black Lives Matter has moved to the center of national attention. The international protests against the police murders of George Floyd and Breonna Taylor and the way the pandemic has exposed how communities of color have borne the brunt of COVID-19 have fueled stunning changes in public opinion about the need for antiracist change.

The pandemic continues to shake our dominant stories and hegemonic stories to their cores, upending our assumptions about what is possible and what is not. When people talk about getting "back to normal," cultural studies teaches us that we are really talking about returning to a familiar story that used to define reality for us. But the pandemic has exposed cracks in old ideas of what normal meant, and especially in all the ways normal proved inadequate to imagining the unimaginable. Or at least how our dominant stories proved inadequate to imagine the future. Other storytellers, from scientists at the Centers for Disease Control and Prevention making projections about the threat of a global pandemic to *The Walking Dead* to Camus's *The Plague* to Steven Soderbergh's *Contagion*, have been thinking about how the world could change in an instant, how a single virus could upend everything we thought we knew and understood.

Before this crisis, racism, income inequality, health care access, climate change, and housing insecurity were already issues. But now we are all experiencing firsthand our desire for new and different answers, for a new and better story of normal to emerge. Cultural studies reminds us that these stories are ours to create and share together. If the stories we have been given are no longer working, it is time for us to reimagine what is possible and tell new ones.

John Alberti is an English professor and cultural studies scholar. He earned his PhD in English from the University of California, Los Angeles. He trusts that stories can facilitate personal and societal transformation. They can motivate us to reevaluate how we do things and our place in the world. Once students grasp the power of stories, then they are able to make critical and empowering observations about the values, ideas, and beliefs embedded in all kinds of stories, from mythology to nursery rhymes, historical narratives to video games. We can all play an active role in interpreting and revising the stories that shape our culture. Alberti's current projects include work on gender in American cinema and television, writing in the digital age, and the movie adaptations of the Harry Potter series.

Embrace the Math You Thought You Would Never Need

Elizabeth McMillan-McCartney

Developmental Mathematics

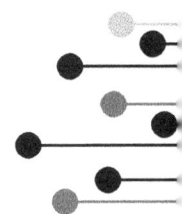

Developmental math courses are designed to help underprepared students learn the basic math, algebra, and critical thinking skills necessary to succeed in their future college-level math courses. A typical complaint from a developmental math student is "When will we ever use this stuff again?" My answer of "You need to be proficient in basic math to take higher-level math classes" does not satisfy. However, more eyes open when I ask students to reflect on encounters outside of class when math has been important.

I encourage any developmental math student to ask, "Where do we encounter mathematics in the COVID-19 pandemic?" Math is useful for understanding the impact of the coronavirus and evaluating our responses to it. Just having a sense of the magnitude of numbers can give more understanding to the trillions of dollars in the stimulus packages, the billions of N95 masks imported, and the millions of people seeking unemployment compensation.

So, what is the difference between a million, a billion, and a trillion? It takes 11.6 days to count to 1 million (assuming one second for each number), about 31.7 years to count to 1 billion, and about 31,700 years to count to 1 trillion. We hear these numbers thrown around so often, yet rarely do we take the time to ponder the staggering differences in scale. By understanding the relative magnitude of these numbers, students are better able to appreciate how long it might take to manufacture 7.8 billion vaccine doses, or one for each person in the world.

Adding, Subtracting, Multiplying, and Dividing
• •

Truly understanding how to add, subtract, multiply, and divide—not mindlessly plugging numbers into a calculator—gives us a powerful thinking tool. For example, repeated multiplication helps us understand exponential growth models. If you multiply a thing by 2 each day, it doubles: 1, 2, 4, 8, 16, 32, 64, 128, and so on. Therefore, a figure of 5,000 COVID-19 cases today increases to 10,000 cases the next day and 640,000 cases just 7 days later. Exponential growth is bad when it comes to the coronavirus. (When it comes to your bank account, exponential growth is reason to celebrate.)

Now you see how the number of coronavirus cases can balloon so quickly when cases are increasing exponentially.

To put the number of COVID-19 cases in context, knowing how to divide numbers can help. When evaluating the extent of the spread of the coronavirus in the United States, it is important to know both the number of cases and the total population of the country (about 330 million). The number of cases is the numerator of the fraction; the total population is the denominator. Note that a denominator can never be zero—that is, no number can be divided by zero. On the other hand, the numerator can be zero, which with COVID-19 cases would be wonderful news—no cases in the population.

At the time of this writing, the number of confirmed cases in the United States is 6,082,260 people (numerator) out of a population of 331 million (denominator). That means there are 0.0184 cases per person. This figure is usually expressed in thousands, or 18.4 cases per 1,000 people. Putting it in terms of rates allows us to compare numbers across populations of unequal size. For example, Italy has 271,515 confirmed cases (numerator) out of a total population of 60 million (denominator). This calculates to 0.0045, or 4.5 cases per 1,000 people. If you subtract the number of cases per 1,000 people of Italy from that of the United States, you will find that the United States has 13.9 more cases per 1,000 people than Italy.[1]

If you are interested in the average (or mean) age of those who have been infected with COVID-19, you must first choose which population you want to examine. Do you want to know the average age of those who have been infected in New York City? The state of Kentucky? The United States? The total number of people who have been infected in your population of interest is the denominator. To calculate an average age, you need to know the age of every individual in that population infected with COVID-19. Then add all the ages together (numerator), and divide by the total number of those infected in your population (denominator).

Until we can test everyone, we can hypothesize that the average will be skewed to an older age range because the most vulnerable (people over age 65) are the most tested. Why? People in older age groups tend to have a weakened immune system and underlying medical conditions, making them more likely to contract the virus and show symptoms, which then prompts them to get tested. If we think the mean is skewed, we might calculate the median, which is a different kind of "average." Finding the median age of those infected requires knowing and listing all their ages, from highest to lowest. The next step is to find the age that falls in the middle of the list, the point at which half of the ages in your list are below that age and half are above that age.[2]

One report from the state of Minnesota showed the median age of known COVID-19 infections as 42 years, and the average age of those who had died as 82 years.[3] CDC data reported that in the entire United States, the median age of people testing positive for COVID-19 was 48. The median age of death was not reported. The CDC report indicated that the most commonly reported ages of death from COVID-19 in the United States are ages over 80 (with or without underlying conditions).

Equations and Formulas

You can think of equations and formulas as a set of steps that you follow to calculate a solution to a problem. Formulas tell you what and when to add, subtract, divide, and multiply. Equations and formulas can help you arrive at solutions for many kinds of COVID-19-related problems. For example, food and grocery delivery drivers would be thankful to receive an appropriate tip—that is, an amount that can be calculated using a suitable percentage.

What tip would you offer for a takeout meal that costs $25.00? If the usual takeout tip is 10%, then multiply the cost of the food ($25.00) by 0.10 (or 10%). Let x equal the amount of the tip and y equal the cost of the food. Mathematicians express the equation this way:

$$x = y * 0.10$$
$$x = \$25.00 * 0.10$$
$$x = \$2.50$$

You can use this formula to calculate a 10% tip for any food price. To be more or less generous, simply adjust the tipping percent up or down, respectively.

As a second example, consider employers who say they will raise essential workers' wages by 5% (or 0.05) during the crisis. Employees earning $10.00 per hour could use the following formula to calculate their new wages, with x equal to the amount of the increase in the current hourly wage and y equal to the current hourly wage:

$$x = y * 0.05$$
$$x = \$10.00 * 0.05$$
$$x = \$0.50$$

Now add $0.50 to the current hourly wage to get the new hourly wage of $10.50. This formula could help workers decide if the increase offered is worth the risk of coming into contact with customers who are potentially infected with the new coronavirus.

Sloping Lines, Ratios, Rates of Change

The idea of "flattening the curve" comes up when the rate of COVID-19 infections is projected to be greater than hospitals can handle. To flatten the curve means to slow the rate down so that fewer people are infected on any given day. Otherwise, too many people may need emergency services at the same time. This danger is why social distancing guidelines were put in place—to keep the medical system from being overwhelmed and to ensure sufficient equipment and other resources to meet the demand for care.

To flatten the curve, the line on a graph showing the number of cases in the population of interest from one day to the next needs to be less steep (or have a smaller slope or rate of change). For instance, if the number of new cases increases by 10 each day (10, 20, 30, 40, 50, etc.), the result is a steeper slope than if the number of new cases increases by 1 each day (1, 2, 3, 4, 5, etc.), which results in a less steep, or flatter, slope.

Researchers who compare COVID-19 data from various countries, including the United States, are interested in the growth factor, the ratio of today's new cases to yesterday's new cases. This number shows how fast the number of new cases is going up or down. If the ratio is greater than 1, then new cases each day are still going up and alarm bells should be ringing. If the ratio is less than 1, then the outbreak is slowing. For example, if today's new cases are 20 and yesterday's new cases were 10, the growth ratio is 20/10 = 2, and the rate of infections are not under control. If, on the other hand, today's new cases are 10 and yesterday's new cases were 20, the growth ratio is 10/20 = 0.5, a much better scenario.

Brush off those algebra notes you thought you would never need. These are just a few examples of how you can use your basic math skills to help make sense of our novel world. It takes more than a calculator. Algebra skills allow you to think in sophisticated ways about an event that is affecting us all. That is the power of math. Math is essential for fighting the coronavirus, for thinking critically and logically about what is happening. It is a vital tool for evaluating the effects of our collective actions, understanding and solving problems, measuring our progress, and figuring out our next steps.

Elizabeth McMillan-McCartney is a senior lecturer emeritus in developmental mathematics. She also taught courses in other levels of mathematics, college orientation, legal research and writing, student advising, and, before her career in teaching, worked in fields that used math modeling and applications. McMillan-McCartney earned degrees in mathematics (BA, Swarthmore College), applied mathematics (MA, Claremont Graduate School, now known as Claremont Graduate University), and law (JD, Salmon P. Chase College of Law). She trusts that math is all around us and that knowledge of addition, subtraction, multiplication, and division can yield critical insights for informing personal choices and policies. The most fundamental rules and concepts of algebra have stood the test of time. Approaching a problem through the lens of mathematics can help us make sense of, and give clarity to, these new situations in which we find ourselves.

Read, Write, Make Meaning

Robert K. Wallace

English Literature

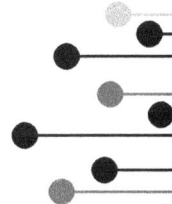

English literature is the study of written works in the English language, including poetry, drama, fiction, nonfiction, and historical documents. A piece of literature is most effective when its author addresses a universal human condition by speaking to, and for, all of us. The discipline of literature encourages people to both read and write. Reading enables us to feel connected to authors. The act of purposely writing with a reader in mind, whether it be for the self (journaling) or someone else, establishes connection.

Reading and writing are meaning-making activities. Enforced periods of social distancing and isolation do not diminish our need to make meaning, and indeed may enhance it. Although discussing works of literature is a highly social act ideally carried out face-to-face, the actual reading and writing are usually intensely private activities that require time for comprehension, composition, and reflection.

When confined to their homes for weeks or months, many people wonder what to do with their time. One way to temporarily escape isolation is to read about the lives of others. Another way is to write. We may not think of ourselves as writers apart from what we have been required to write in school or at work. But we can look to ourselves and others we know, or have known, to find subject material. Informal personal writing can be therapeutic. Such writing can also be meaningful to those with whom it is shared.

One of the simplest examples that the value of informal writing can bring is an assignment often given to schoolchildren: Make a card with a written message to a loved one saying how you love or care for them. Doing so enriches the child who writes it, as well as the recipient who reads it.

A more sophisticated example of self-expression and shared experience is the published autobiography written by Frederick Douglass. Few have a life story as compelling or urgent as his. Douglass published his first autobiography, *Narrative of the Life of Frederick Douglass, an American Slave*, in 1845, seven years after his escape from slavery.[1] He wrote his narrative for himself as well as for others.

During times of enforced isolation, as with the COVID-19 crisis, anyone could benefit from reading Douglass's *Narrative*. The story is relatively short (about 100 pages), and the language is direct and easily accessible. The narrative voice is authentic and trustworthy. I find that this book appeals to first-year students in a general studies course as much as it does to upper-division

English majors. It appeals equally to people of all ethnic groups and nations. Any reader can admire the way young Douglass overcomes one struggle after another, continuing to find faith in the face of trauma and oppression.

How might readers who find themselves in food lines or unable to pay rent find relevance in Douglass's *Narrative* and the goal he had of writing for the benefit of others? And how might readers today use Douglass as a model for writing about their own lives, to enrich their lives or those of others?

Douglass published *Narrative* to prove he had actually been enslaved (he spoke so eloquently that many had doubted this). When he escaped enslavement in Maryland in 1838 and arrived in New Bedford, Massachusetts, he took the name of Douglass to make it harder for slaveholders who knew him as Frederick Bailey to find him. By writing *Narrative*, he outed himself and his owners by using their true names. But in doing so, he endangered himself, because those owners could have learned of his whereabouts. If they had come to claim him, state authorities would have been legally compelled under the Fugitive Slave Law to send him back. For that reason, several months after the book was published, Douglass left for a two-year lecture tour of Great Britain, returning only after supporters there had purchased his freedom.

Douglass's overriding goal in *Narrative* was to convey to Americans, especially in the North, the reality of slavery in the South. He emphasized the damage slavery did to the heart, mind, and soul of its victims even more than the damage done to the physical body through whipping, torture, and cold-blooded murder. As he wrote, he discovered surprising things about himself as well as others. Although he wrote the book to convey slavery's reality to readers, much of the knowledge conveyed grew out of the process of writing itself.

For instance, when Douglass was enslaved, he did not understand the meaning or purpose of the strange songs that groups of enslaved persons sang when marching to the master's house. In writing about these songs of freedom, he realized that "they told a tale" in "tone loud, long, and deep; they breathed the prayer and complaint of souls boiling over with the bitterest anguish." He came to understand that "slaves sing most when they are most unhappy. The songs of the slave represent the sorrows of his heart; and he is relieved by them, only as an aching heart is relieved by its tears." This passage appears to be the first time anyone had ever written about the musical, psychological, and communal value of the songs of the enslaved that still move us so much today. Douglass confessed, as he was writing the passage, that a tear had "already found its way down my cheek."

Douglass also recalled Mrs. Auld, the first white person who had ever looked on him with kindness. Mrs. Auld taught Douglass to read. "The frequent hearing of my mistress reading the bible—for she often read aloud when her husband was absent—soon awakened my curiosity in respect to this mystery of reading, and roused in me the desire to learn. Having no fear of my kind mistress before my eyes (she had given me no reason to fear),

I frankly asked her to teach me to read; and without hesitation, the dear woman began the task, and very soon, by her assistance, I was master of the alphabet, and could spell words of three or four letters."

As soon as Hugh Auld realized his wife was teaching young Frederick to read, he stopped her, "telling her, in the first place, that the thing itself was unlawful; that it was also unsafe, and could only lead to mischief." Young Douglass was bitterly disappointed at the time, but Mr. Auld's intervention taught him, as nothing else could, that learning to read must be very valuable if his master had worked to prevent it. Reading and writing became Douglass's "pathway to freedom." Writing about this enabled Douglass to share this realization with the reader. When Mrs. Auld changed for the worse after she could no longer teach him, Douglass realized how much slavery diminished the humanity of the slaveholders themselves.

Reading Douglass's account of learning to read calls to mind the millions of elementary students reading at home instead of in school because of COVID-19. How many of them have someone like Mrs. Auld, who had once cared for Frederick and helped him to read and form his words? And if they do not, how many have someone like Mr. Auld, who, in seeking to undermine their efforts to read, spurs them on? And what about children for whom no one notices or cares that they learn to read?

Douglass reached a low point in his life after being farmed out to the slave breaker Edward Covey. Covey abused him physically and psychologically until young Frederick's "natural elasticity was crushed." It was then that young Douglass recalled the "white sails" of the large ships that would sail past him on Chesapeake Bay. These sails were free and in motion, whereas he was enslaved and confined. But watching them sail past gave him an image of freedom he could aspire to. "O that I were free! O, that I were on one of your gallant decks, and under your protecting wing! Alas! Betwixt me and you, the turbid waters roll. Go on, go on. O that I could also go!" Soon after this passage in which his spirit was freed, Douglass shows us the inner strength that inspired him to fight back when Covey attacked him during the battle in which he as a "slave became a man."

When young Douglass finally escaped to freedom in New York City, he was not as free as he expected. Slave catchers were swarming the city, eager to make quick money by capturing and turning over a fugitive like him. Only the generosity of David Ruggles, a Black New Yorker who ran the Underground Railroad in the city, saved him from an uncertain fate. It was through the kindness of this total stranger that Douglass and his wife, Anna, made it to the relatively safe haven of New Bedford. Douglass describes a fugitive as one who is "without home or friends—without money or credit—wanting shelter, and no one to give it—wanting bread, and no money to buy it."

In this condition, he is "pursued by merciless men-hunters, and in total darkness as to what to do, where to go, or where to stay—perfectly helpless both as to the means of defense and means of escape—in the midst of plenty, yet suffering the terrible gnawings of hunger—in the midst of houses, yet having no home." Douglass's words resonate with those who are enduring hardship, who are hungry, who are pursued, or who find themselves in any helpless condition.

Why would it be good to read Douglass's *Narrative* in the isolation of the coronavirus pandemic? First, for the inspiring story of a person who overcame seemingly insurmountable obstacles. This pandemic is especially frightening because we cannot predict when it will end. Just as Douglass hoped enslavement would end, we also can hope that the current pandemic will end or diminish.

Reading the *Narrative of the Life of Frederick Douglass* can be instructive in a time like ours because his words enable us to empathize in the pain of others while also strengthening our own inner resolve. But perhaps even more therapeutic is the process of writing our own narratives for ourselves or for others. Many of us rely on phones and the Internet to communicate with people we know and love in times of self-isolation, but writing to them takes our thoughts and feelings to a deeper, more permanent layer of expression.

During times of crisis, such as with the COVID-19 pandemic, reading and writing can be valuable for exploring ourselves and making us more grateful for the experiences and human connections that have enriched us. Consider also that what we discover about ourselves can be good to share with others, who will appreciate reading about what they have done to make a positive difference in our life. To create personal writing exercises, we can ask ourselves the following kinds of questions:

> What would you like to write to a grandparent, parent, sibling, friend, or fellow employee that you have never made the time to say?

> What sacrifice have loved ones made for you that you would like to acknowledge in writing?

> Are there people who have intervened in your life to make it better, to whom you might write to express your thanks?

> Have you had an encounter with an Edward Covey, a Mr. Auld, or a Mrs. Auld that you could sort through by writing?

Those of us who have the time and space can use reading and personal writing to expand our horizons, explore and focus our feelings, and make meaning of this pandemic and the effects it has had on our lives, both individually and communally.

Robert K. Wallace is a Regents Professor of English. He teaches Frederick Douglass to a first-year writing course called Exploring the Arts and to upper-division students in the course Frederick Douglass and Cincinnati Antislavery. He earned his PhD in English from Columbia University. Wallace trusts in the efficacy of

Douglass as a writer because of the directness of his Narrative and its universal appeal. When he asks first-year students whether they see the Narrative more as a historical document or something that speaks to us today, most say both. Yes, this book does help them to see what slavery was like in the 19th century, but Douglass's book also speaks to their own educational aspirations, to the need they see for mutual understanding among different racial and ethnic groups, and to their desire to address pressing national needs. They feel through Douglass the need to know our history to face the future.

Don't Blame the Bats

Jaime McCauley

Environmental Sociology

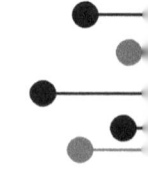

More than a third of the world's population faced some type of restriction on movement in an effort to stop the spread of the coronavirus. As increasing numbers of people were ordered to stay at home, interactions between people dropped dramatically as highways cleared and flights were grounded. Shops and restaurants shuttered. Busy tourist destinations stood eerily empty.

With these changes, we saw something new in social media: photos celebrating noticeable improvements to air and water quality in the absence of pollution. We saw a smog-free Los Angeles skyline and Himalayan mountain peaks visible from India (for the first time in almost 30 years). Hitting pause on the fast-paced, round-the-clock culture of our postmodern world made painfully clear the degree to which human activity has harmed the environment.

Environmental sociologists examine the adverse impact that this high level of human activity has on the environment, especially on air and water quality. They also examine the ways this environmental deterioration ricochets back to harm us, often in unequal ways. As the saying goes: What we do to Earth, we do to ourselves.

When we think of harm to the environment, we typically think of harm caused by material by-products (chemicals, toxins, and other hazardous waste) that modern industrial life spews into the environment, contaminating air, soil, and water. While humans have always interacted with and manipulated the environments in which we live, as all organisms do, our impact has grown exponentially since the dawn of the industrial age, which began around 1750, with the most rapid changes occurring since the mid-1950s. Without a doubt, industrial and technological advancements have improved the life expectancy and quality of life for most humans around the globe. However, these advancements have a dark side.

The population of Earth now exceeds 7 billion people. Accommodating modern consumer demands and human population growth strains the natural environment, including nonhuman species. Environmental change on this scale simply cannot take place without concurrently changing human and animal life, health, and interaction.

Specifically, we do not consider how the social and economic changes that came with industrialization result in stresses on human and nonhuman species. These changes created the conditions that made it easier for the novel coronavirus to be transmitted from animals to humans and to move rapidly across populations. These efficient modes of transmission fuel epidemic and pandemic episodes, leaving humans vulnerable. And some humans are more vulnerable than others.

Poor air quality associated with traffic congestion, industrial outputs, and burning fossil fuels is linked to higher rates of asthma, lung diseases, reduced pulmonary function, and cancer. Because COVID-19 attacks lung function, people living with poor air quality are at higher risk for long recovery times or death.

Environmental inequality generally refers to the unequal distribution of environmental "goods" (access to public parks and green space, clean air and water) and "bads" (poor air quality, proximity to toxic dumping, noise pollution). Environmental racism refers to the ways in which communities of color specifically are subject to a disproportionate amount of environmental bads. Both of these concepts overlay the experience of illness and death in our modern pandemics, including that of COVID-19.[1]

Epidemics and pandemics are not new in human history. However, the level of vulnerability has deepened. Another driver of modern pandemics is the loss of animal habitat and biodiversity. Most notably, humans and their industrial and agricultural enterprises encroach on wildlife habitats, forcing animals into human spaces. Increased potential for interaction puts wildlife on a collision course with humans, creating opportunities for zoonotic infection (i.e., transmission of viruses from animals to humans). While zoonotic virus transmission is not new, industrialization, urbanization, globalization, and their associated economic, cultural, and demographic changes create conditions for zoonotic illnesses to reach pandemic proportions.[2] Habitat loss is so extensive that many scientists fear we are in the midst of a mass extinction event.[3] By one estimate, 28,000 species are threatened with extinction, 24,000 of which are threatened by agricultural expansion.[4]

Recent pandemics underscore the link between humans and animals. AIDS, Ebola, H1N1 (swine flu), SARS, and COVID-19 are all illnesses first transmitted to the human population via interaction with animals. The best known and most extensively researched of pandemics is HIV/AIDS.

The start of the modern AIDS pandemic is typically traced back to the early 1980s. In the decades that followed, HIV/AIDS claimed the lives of 25 million people around the world, and 30 million people are currently HIV positive. The roots of this modern pandemic illustrate how industrialization, urbanization, and globalization can collectively fuel an outbreak. The viral host of HIV is understood to be a certain species of chimpanzees hunted for food or ritual purposes in parts of central Africa, with the virus transmitted to humans during the butchering process.[5]

Isolated cases of what we now call HIV/AIDS no doubt occurred in humans over an untold period of time. The infection rate changed, however, when Belgian colonizers cleared central African land for mining, logging, and extraction of other raw materials to set up the region as a supplier of raw goods, dramatically changing economic and cultural life.

The virus was then spread via sexual contact and unsterilized hypodermic needles used in vaccination campaigns. By the 1960s, most Belgian colonists had returned to Europe, no doubt taking some AIDS cases with them. Later, Haitian migrant workers traveled to central Africa. When these workers left in the late 1970s, they likely took a few cases with them as well. These few isolated clusters of illness drew little attention, but by the 1980s, globalization was now fully underway. A pandemic was born.[6]

There is less certainty around the origin and transmission of Ebola virus, though it, too, is likely transmitted when handling infected "bushmeat." The virus's main carrier is thought to be bats, which transmit the virus to other animals through blood or bodily fluids. Human transmission occurs when an infected chimpanzee, antelope, porcupine, or other animal is prepared for consumption. While the first case of Ebola was recorded in 1976, isolated cases no doubt existed prior.

Between the 1970s and 2000s, global demand for raw materials pushed humans to encroach further into African territory, and with them came increased human population density, destruction of habitat, and other anthropogenic disturbances. These factors set the stage for what would become the deadliest recorded outbreak of Ebola from 2014 to 2016. Rooted in environmental disruption and fueled by global travel, more than 11,000 people died from Ebola virus disease.[7,8]

Research on coronavirus illnesses (SARS and COVID-19) illustrates the delicate connections between environmental degradation, zoonotic virus transmission, and pandemic potential. Bats are believed to host the new coronavirus but not transmit it directly to humans. There is some evidence that intermediate hosts are involved. Likely candidates include civets and pangolins—two prized species traded on the exotic animal market. Keeping these animals in captivity increases the odds of humans contracting the virus.[9] Moreover, China has undergone a period of rapid industrialization, urbanization, and economic growth. In the process, the balance of animal–human interaction has changed a great deal. Not only are animal–human "crossings" more likely than ever before, but a growing middle class means more people have an opportunity to purchase exotic animals—some of which are known to carry coronaviruses.[10,11,12]

It is not the bat's fault. Or the chimps, or civets, or pangolins. Animals are living the lives they have always led, minding their own business. We are the ones encroaching on their territory, butchering them or selling them in markets, destroying habitats, and restructuring the balance of the environment. While animals may play a role in disease transmission, human activity is the driving force behind the growth in virus transmission.

When reports emerged of clearer air, cleaner water, and animals frolicking in deserted city streets around the world, an Internet meme arose stating: "We are the virus." This meme was meant to underscore the belief that nature could heal itself if only humans stayed out of the way. This take is not entirely wrong. Humans have indeed caused a great deal of damage to Earth. However, the story does not end there. The problem is that humans are not separate from the environment; we are part of it. Thinking that humans should just get out of the way does not account for who is doing the most damage[13] and will only prolong our inaction on real environmental change.

Jaime McCauley is an associate professor of sociology at Coastal Carolina University and earned her PhD from the University of Windsor (Ontario, Canada). She trusts the idea presented in this paper because the impact of 7 billion people and their related survival needs and consumer demands has caused tremendous change to human–animal interactions and relationships. It is only natural that change at this scale comes at some risk to human populations and, in addition, inflicts harm on nonhuman species.

See the Predictability in the Chaos of Pandemics

Tom Zaniello

Film Studies

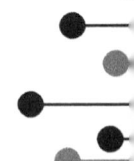

S tudents who take courses in film studies explore many topics, including the art and techniques of storytelling, genre, film theory, film history, and of course, filmmaking. Here we examine a specific genre of film—epidemic cinema—that informs popular understanding of pandemics, and specifically, our understanding of the COVID-19 pandemic.

It goes without saying that epidemic cinema features an epidemic or a pandemic.[1] Epidemic cinema gives us imagery and narrative about pandemics that shape the public's perception of infectious diseases, how they came to be, and how they move through populations. These films are not invested in depicting an accurate account of the biology of viruses. They do, however, focus on all that can go wrong with the spread of viruses. In this sense, the chaos in the films mirrors the chaos of real pandemics. Studying the epidemic genre helps us see some of the predictability in the chaos.

Epidemic cinema gives attention to how a virus or other disease vector leads to a breakdown in the social order and in institutions. These films give viewers an opportunity to identify with characters like themselves, faced with overwhelming anxieties fueled by the prospect of a dangerous future. Epidemic cinema shows how the public is at the mercy of heroic and devious medical professionals, government officials, and military forces. Every film tracks the development of the pandemic from its first victims to widespread contamination while governments scramble to alleviate the inevitable "panic in the streets."[2] After showing how the pandemic radically reorganizes the social order, the films offer resolutions that range from the reassuring to the terrifying.

Below is a checklist of epidemic cinema indicators, adapted and expanded from the Williamson-Finch paradigm.[3] These indicators are important because they reveal narrative patterns that make predictable what seems unknowable in pandemics.

- ✓ What is the contagious disease in the film?
- ✓ Is the disease vector bacterial, viral, fungal, protozoan, inorganic, or a natural force?
- ✓ Are there mutations or unpredictable changes in the vector?
- ✓ When and where is the pandemic believed to have started?

✓ How are "blood imagery," "body horrors," and other bodily fluids revealed?

✓ What crimes are observed during the pandemic?

✓ Are foreigners, immigrants, and ethnic or racial minorities targeted?

✓ Is the white middle-class family idealized in the film?

✓ What roles do medical personnel, police, and military have in combating the pandemic?

✓ How does the pharmaceutical industry intervene?

✓ How do "government indifference, conspiracy, or disbelief" augment the pandemic?

✓ Is a "Patient Zero" or a "superspreader" of the disease identified?

✓ Who gets quarantined, and why?

✓ Are infected nonhuman "species," such as zombies, central to the plot?

✓ Has a postapocalyptic society or a new order prevailed?

This checklist of indicators draws attention to the patterns in every pandemic film and serves as a guide for thinking through the dynamics of real-life pandemics. The examination of specific pandemic films and documentaries,[4] such as those discussed in this idea paper, are also instructive.

Kazan's film *Panic in the Streets* (1950) is set in New Orleans during an outbreak of bubonic plague. Among the working class and lumpenproletariat (criminals) is Patient Zero, a victim of bubonic plague bacteria and an undocumented immigrant concealed by a criminal underworld of fellow immigrants and precarious workers. The ship that has smuggled him in is staffed by a Black and Asian crew portrayed as un-American. Three men rob Patient Zero and kill him. The murderers contract bubonic plague but do not realize it. The police rush to locate and capture the murderers because anyone the dead man has contact with will die within 48 hours without a serum inoculation. Like *Panic in the Streets*, during the coronavirus crisis we have confronted anti-immigrant claims that the COVID-19 pathogen is a "Chinese virus," a claim that motivated some to target, harass, and attack people in the Asian category. Related claims include the Chinese rebuttal that the U.S. military brought the virus to Wuhan.

The film *The Andromeda Strain* (1971/2008)[5] demonstrates the mise-en-scène[6] of epidemic cinema. In the first sequence, men in body-protective suits arrive in a remote town in which everyone—except a crying infant and an alcoholic old man—is dead, their bodies devoid of blood, which has been replaced by what seems to be powder. Investigators eventually determine that the victims have died of a crystalline virus originating from outer space. Through medical sleuthing the disease vector is exposed, and in the process, the U.S. government is found responsible for probing outer space for such a pathogen to use as a biochemical weapon. This kind of conspiracy runs through a number of epidemic films. Some well-known conspiracy theories that have circulated around COVID-19 include one that claims that the new coronavirus is a biological weapon spread more quickly by the introduction of 5G networks.

The TV series *Containment* (2016) involves epidemic pathogens and investigators who make numerous false steps, causing panic in their community. The competition between medical staff and police forces in the quest for isolating Patient Zero also contributes to the difficulty in controlling the epidemic. In the show, a whole district of Atlanta must be sealed off by a giant barrier wall of shipping containers to keep those possibly infected from entering the city's general population. In our present COVID-19 crisis, the state authority to prevent travelers from crossing borders has become a contentious issue. If shows and films are any guide, failing to clarify state authority in a timely manner can lead to regional crises and a loss of faith in the government to contain the virus.

Still another intriguing set of variations of the pathogen and its transmittance through human populations is offered in *Outbreak* (1995). A fictional virus called "Motaba," a variation of the Ebola virus, attacks a village in Zaire, which the American Air Force subsequently obliterates to contain the virus.[7] It becomes apparent, however, that an infected monkey from Zaire has been smuggled into the United States for commercial sale. The monkey escapes its cage and is seen darting about a suburban backyard where a child is playing. The American military plans to bomb the suburban community in an attempt to control the spread of the virus once again. Eventually, it is revealed that the military leadership has been in search of a pathogen to use for its own chemical–biological arsenal.

Outbreak warns viewers about the power misused and misapplied during the coronavirus pandemic. In the name of controlling the virus or out of motivation to underplay the depth of the crisis, concerns about personal freedoms, privacy, and safety are at high risk of being brushed aside. Until May 6, 2020, several months into the pandemic, the country undercounted COVID-19 cases and deaths because the Centers for Disease Control and Prevention did not require nursing homes to report them. In addition to playing down COVID-19's toll, the underreporting resulted in slowing the response for protecting this population and the health care workers who serve them.

The Leakers (2018), a Hong Kong-based epidemic thriller, offers lessons about how powerful players such as pharmaceutical companies and medical health care suppliers can shape the course of events during a pandemic. In this film, the CEO of a pharmaceutical company has engineered both a mosquito-borne Zika virus and its vaccine, with a plan to release the virus and sell the cure. The lesson is that the circumstances of a pandemic can provide ample economic opportunity for the players involved in its management. For example, with COVID-19, when the federal government ordered states to purchase their own ventilators and other medical supplies, the stage was set for a bidding war pitting states against each other and ultimately benefiting the suppliers. Ventilators jumped in cost from $25,000 to $40,000 a unit.[8]

The Killer That Stalked New York is a melodramatic film noir made in 1950. The killer is a criminal, a woman arriving from Cuba with $50,000 in diamonds to sell, but she is also infected with smallpox. The police are worried about the diamonds, but medical detectives are more concerned about the virus. The people of New York City begin to receive inoculations, but there are not enough vaccines for 8 million. Panic hits the streets. Neighborhood police stations are turned into clinics and eventually the virus is contained. "Forced back," a medical officer says, "to the Middle Ages where it belonged."

Issues around vaccine shortages also apply to the COVID-19 crisis. When the vaccine is finally produced, will there be enough to go around? And how will it be distributed? Epidemic cinema warns us that we will be unprepared unless we are able to produce not only a sufficient amount of vaccine but also the medical supplies needed to package and administer it. Also needed is a logical and equitable plan for whom and how it will be distributed as it is produced.

The documentary *Cooked: Survival by Zip Code* (2019) chronicles an unusual kind of epidemic, the little-known heat wave that hit Chicago in 1995. During five days in July, daily temperatures reached 100 degrees or higher, causing 739 people, mostly African Americans, to die of heat-related causes. Most were afraid or unable to leave their un-air-conditioned apartments, even reluctant to open their windows for fear of robbery. The disease vector here was extreme heat; the preexisting conditions were poverty and ill health. Other preexisting social inequalities that contribute to a pandemic are unemployment, foreclosure, inadequate food markets, crime, incarceration, gun violence, and vacant buildings and lots. In both the film and the COVID-19 pandemic, refrigerated trailer trucks were parked in the lots of Chicago hospitals to serve as portable morgues. COVID-19's disproportionate impact on the African American population because of underlying medical conditions, inadequate medical care, and centuries of discrimination might have been less harsh if the lessons of *Cooked* had been minded.

Now we turn to the first two films that deal explicitly with the COVID-19 pandemic, both made in the early stages of the virus's spread. The first is Naomi Klein's short film *Corona Capitalism—And How to Beat It*. Klein is a social activist who critiques capitalism in general and corona-related capitalism in a nine-minute agit-prop[9] documentary, an analytical attack on the American ruling elite and businessmen "using the disaster as a cover for capitalist expansion." Klein warns us that during crises, political agendas and the profit-taking excesses of capitalism are revealed. "We know this script," she argues. "All the most dangerous ideas lying around, from privatizing Social Security to locking down borders to caging even more migrants" can be advanced during a crisis. The point of the film is that leaders in the highest places use the cover of crisis to quickly pass legislation and make executive orders without the normal checks and balances.

In the second film, Mostafa Keshvari's scripted feature *Corona*, seven people are trapped in an apartment house elevator. The passengers are a cross-section of Middle America: a pregnant white woman, a Black elevator repairman, a white woman used to being listened to, a white man who uses a wheelchair and has a swastika tattooed on his forehead, one of the building owners, and a tenant in debt. The last to enter the elevator is a Chinese Canadian woman who coughs just before the elevator stops moving. When she coughs, it is clear everyone else believes she is ill with COVID-19. When the elevator stalls, red emergency lights begin flashing, and the man with the swastika tattoo takes out a gun. We hear a scream: "We're all going to die in here!" Another shouts: "We're all being tested here." The profound conclusion stated earlier in the trailer for the film is that "fear is a virus."

Why are these films important for us to view during the COVID-19 pandemic? Because they use a pandemic as a metaphor for social breakdown and political collapse. They serve as a warning about what can go wrong in a real pandemic.[10] Epidemics reveal disproportionate harm to the vulnerable and marginalized. Quarantine exacerbates stigma and discrimination. And travel bans amplify xenophobia. These films warn against becoming sidetracked by conspiracy theories (the "plandemic" to bring down President Trump), denial (does the virus even exist?), or indifference (the oldest adults, who are among the most vulnerable, are about to die of something soon anyway).

Seven years ago, David Quammen, author of *Spillover: Animal Infections and the Next Human Pandemic,* wrote a *New York Times* op-ed column titled "The Next Pandemic: Not If, but When." He wrote that coronaviruses are dangerous because of "their high rates of mutation and their proclivity for recombination." He concluded that "one emergent virus, sooner or later, will be the Next Big One." He was right, and studying epidemic cinema will perhaps guide us in responding to the COVID-19 crisis and in making us more attentive and proactive with the next pandemic.

Tom Zaniello earned his PhD from Stanford University. He is an emeritus professor and taught film studies and honors courses in epidemic cinema and catastrophes. He has programmed film festivals on labor and other topics in Washington, DC, London, and Liverpool. His book The Cinema of the Precariat: The Exploited, Underemployed, and Temp Workers of the World *(2020) includes a chapter on epidemic cinema and catastrophic mise-en-scène. Zaniello trusts the checklist of indicators presented in this paper because they are a synthesis of patterns observed and gathered from teaching and viewing more than 50 films about epidemics.*

Behave as if You Are Contagious

Linda Dynan

Health Economics

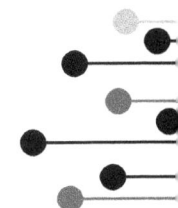

Economists study relationships among consumers, sellers, and others involved in producing, purchasing, and consuming market and nonmarket goods and services. They understand that the individual choices people make, whatever their role in an economic decision, add up to impact economies and entire societies. Economists assume that choices are made under conditions of scarcity rooted in the imbalance between the limitless wants of consumers and the limited resources of sellers.

A perfectly competitive market offsets this imbalance between wants and resources. Economists have identified the conditions (listed in no particular order) of a perfectly competitive market:

1. There are many buyers and sellers to ensure healthy competition.

2. Sellers can freely enter the market (begin selling product) and exit the market (stop selling product).

3. Buyers have complete information about the price and quality of the product being sold.

4. Sellers are selling identical products.[1]

In reality, perfect markets do not exist.[2] But the more a market departs from these conditions, the less economically and socially optimal are the outcomes. Some problems of imbalance include market-dominating firms having the power to set prices above the worth of their products or to set prices low enough to drive out other sellers; uninformed consumers being unable to serve as a check on quality and price; and people with less income not being able to afford the purchase of products and services.

Health Care Markets

Because health care markets are not perfectly competitive, the health care system in the United States is highly vulnerable in normal times. It is even more so in times of crisis. Why is this? Because the health care market is an extreme example of *not* meeting any of the four conditions.

First, many parts of the country have very few health care providers or sellers. In many places there is no hospital or only one hospital. In other areas, a hospital system dominates the region (Condition 1). One reason for this circumstance is that it is extremely difficult for health care providers to enter and exit the market because of the numerous rules and regulations (Condition 2). Consumers cannot freely enter into a hospital or doctor's office because often they do not know what they need[3] or what the visit will cost. And although insurance companies are in place to offset the financial risk, consumers are never sure how much of their total cost will be covered (Condition 3).[4]

Finally, health care is also not easily shoppable. It is difficult to compare the price and quality of services among providers and sellers. To further complicate matters, often a set of services comes with each episode of care, such as with a knee replacement, that makes comparison shopping more complex. A consumer might wonder if two different hospitals perform a knee replacement surgery in the same way. Do the hospitals offer identical "products," and what is the cost for each? If the sets of services are different, then knowing their cost is not entirely useful for the consumer. (It is like comparing apples to oranges.) The same questions can be asked about a visit to the doctor (Condition 4).

Additionally, consider that people do not purchase services and products only from doctors and hospitals. We buy a variety of health care products on the market that we believe will enhance our health, such as gym memberships and nutritious foods. People also engage in behaviors known to reduce good health, such as smoking or excessive drinking. To further complicate matters, our health can be impacted by choices that we do not make ourselves and are a result of the choices of others. Economists call a behavior of others that affects us unfavorably a *negative externality*. A negative externality puts the costs on the person who was adversely impacted by that negligent behavior. For example, the cost of secondhand smoke to a person's health is not paid for by the smoker.[5]

The transmission of COVID-19 is also a negative externality. The illness is highly contagious, easily transmitted through normal human actions (face touching) and interactions (hanging out with friends), and the virus that causes it can be spread by asymptomatic people.[6] The coronavirus pandemic adds more uncertainty to already existing vulnerabilities in health care. It presents an especially dangerous health care crisis because it is fueled by negligent, careless, and uninformed behaviors such as interacting without wearing a mask and not practicing social distancing. These seemingly benign behaviors have far-reaching effects on others and the health care system.

Fortunately, people can and do change their behavior to prevent becoming ill. Examples are condom use for HIV/AIDS prevention and hand washing during cold and flu season. Such changes may be motivated by self-interest, the penalty of law, or the desire to be a good citizen. However, when individuals do not bear the full burden of their behaviors, a government can create laws and incentives through taxes, subsidies, price controls, rationing, quarantines, mandated social distancing, and required or recommended use of protective equipment, such as masks, to change those individual behaviors so that individual choice and societal well-being converge. Although government intervention may interfere with perfectly competitive conditions, it is likely to improve outcomes when individuals do not choose to take responsibility for the effects of their own behaviors on others.

Social Distancing as Collective Action

Engaging in collective action does not come naturally. Individuals tend to think and act in terms of pursuing their own interest rather than the collective interest. To get through this health care crisis, everyone must participate in collective action aimed at reducing transmission. The extent to which social distancing effectively reduces the number of COVID-19 cases depends on community-wide participation. Given that in most situations it is impossible to determine who is contagious, everyone must behave as though they are.

Failure to take preventative measures inevitably increases the number of infected people turning to health care and leads to the system becoming overwhelmed. Ultimately, making an investment in social distancing is about protecting our fragile health care system. When the demand is such that hospitals are inundated with patients, medical staff must expend time and energy to confront ethical dilemmas related to supply, including how to allocate limited resources. Who gets an ICU bed? Who gets personal protective equipment? Who can visit their sick or dying relatives? What about people not infected with the coronavirus who require emergency care? This frightening situation illustrates vividly how private actions and societal well-being must meet.

Until we produce a vaccine, we know that social distancing is the most effective way to contain and mitigate the risks of contracting the virus and becoming sick with COVID-19. Ironically, even though social distancing comes at a high personal and economic cost, it is necessary for ultimate economic survival. Every business and organization that draws crowds must find creative ways to sell its services and products while keeping customers safe. And remember to do your part—act as though you are contagious as you move about in the world. Think of your behavior as an investment—in your own health, others' health, and in the health of our health care system.

Linda Dynan is a health economist and professor of economics who earned her PhD in economics from Columbia University. Dynan's research interests and grant writing focus on health economics. She completed her postdoctoral studies as a Crosby Research Fellow with the Hospital Research and Educational Trust of the American Hospital Association. She trusts in conditions of perfect competition because when the principles are violated in practice, it is well documented that problems arise.

Discover a Blueprint to See a Way Out

William Landon

History

Historians study, record, and interpret events that happened in the past. Depending on the point of view they employ, historians also reinterpret and amend history in light of new information. They take care to place historical events in the context of social, religious, economic, and political forces shaping life at that particular time and place. When historians are asked about a current event[1] such as this novel coronavirus pandemic, they contextualize what they are seeing within the history of previous pandemics that the world has faced.

To understand and tackle this present pandemic, historical knowledge is essential not only for historians but also for epidemiologists, virologists, and pharmacologists, who have their own history and historians. These disciplines draw on historical thinking to examine how humanity reacted to and overcame previous pandemics, including which restrictions and treatments were most effective. When navigating tumultuous waters, knowledge of the past helps us to gain our bearings.

Every historian asks: Has the world faced an event such as this before? The answer here is a resounding "yes." In fact, it has faced a number of pandemics. Take a moment to reflect upon the past 102 years (1918–2020). During this relatively short span of human history, there has been SARS, MERS, Ebola, and H1N1. The mortality for each of these four viruses was less than 15,000 worldwide, a number that pales in comparison to the ongoing HIV/AIDS pandemic (30 million deaths worldwide), the ever-present mosquito-borne malaria (450,000 deaths), and seasonally recurring outbreaks of influenza (291,000–646,000 deaths worldwide per year). The worldwide toll brought about by the 1918–1920 influenza pandemic (caused by an H1N1 virus) resulted in 500 million infections and 50 million deaths.[2]

As we face the COVID-19 pandemic, there is the very real sense that what is already a situation of the gravest concern will certainly get worse. At the time of this writing, there were 25.8 million confirmed cases globally and 858,072 deaths (if you go to the URL in this endnote, you will see the most recent numbers available).[3]

Like many of you reading this, I have been working from home since my university moved all our instruction to an online format. This necessary change allowed me to invest my time in reflecting on this question: What does history have to teach us about our present circumstances? Using the lens of history, I read news from around the world (and locally) voraciously. The patterns in human responses to this pandemic are interesting.

It has become clear to me that despite advancements in technology and communication, we as a species have not changed much since 1347–1351, when the Black Death, the most fatal pandemic recorded in human history, struck Italy and then all of Europe, killing an estimated 75 million to 200 million people. Called the Black Death because of its signature symptom of black growths, called buboes, that erupted from lymph nodes in the armpit, groin, and neck, it was a combination of bubonic, septicemic, and pneumonic plagues.[4]

The Black Death pathogen, like that of COVID-19, was transmitted from animals to humans and spread locally, regionally, nationally, and globally as a result of trade and the movement of goods and people. The cause of both COVID-19 and the Black Death is zoonotic, meaning that the disease agent originated in nonhuman animal hosts. (The virus that causes COVID-19 is believed to have originated in bats.)[5]

In the case of the Black Death, the infectious bacterium populated rodents, specifically the rat (*Rattus norvegicus*). Fleas that bit infected rodents to feed off their blood acquired the bacteria. When a rat host perished from the plague (yes, rats and wild and domesticated animals also died from the disease), epidemiologists believe that parasitic fleas, which carried the plague bacteria in their gut, sought new hosts—humans. Infected humans then passed the deadly bacteria on to fellow humans via bodily fluids. In densely populated European cities, where sanitation and personal hygiene were often neglected completely, it was only a matter of time before hot spots of infection developed. And, as a result of trade between European regions, these hot spots eventually covered the continent.

A historical text written during the Black Death resonates deeply with current events—Giovanni Boccaccio's *The Decameron*. Each page is informed by the first and largest medieval outbreak. *The Decameron* is a truly great piece of literature because it transcends the time in which it was written, often speaking directly to our present situation and providing guidance from our collective past.[6] If you have not read this text, some background is useful. The prologue contains the most famous description of the transmission of the plague and the devastation it caused; we need to consider it now, if we are to understand our responses to COVID-19.

Boccaccio writes: "And the plague gathered strength as it was transmitted from the sick to the healthy through normal intercourse, just as fire catches on to any dry or greasy object placed too close to it. Nor did it stop there: not only did the healthy incur the disease and with it the prevailing mortality by talking to or keeping company with the sick—they had only to touch the clothing or anything else that had come into contact with or been used by the sick and the plague evidently was passed to the one who handled those things."

Responses to the Black Death

As a result of firsthand observation, Boccaccio divided human responses to the plague into four distinct categories. Described are, according to the Italian writer, the four fundamental ways that people reacted to the plague.

Sheltering in Place. Sometimes people sheltered in place with a small group of family and friends. Boccaccio noted that this group included those who remained in the city and took care not to heed the horrific sounds outside their doors. They ate and drank temperately and did their best to while away the time playing music, singing, and conversing with one another.

Overindulging in Every Form of Physical Pleasure. This category includes the people who gathered in large groups and set about living what was left of life to the fullest: tramping from tavern to tavern, drinking, singing, copulating, and otherwise indulging. Obviously, making such a response to life during a plague made it difficult to avoid those who were sick and those whose symptoms had not yet presented.

Maintaining Daily Routines. These are the people who walked around the city trying to work, avoiding the sick and covering their faces with handkerchiefs filled with herbs whenever they passed through the streets. The herbs were the antidote to "bad air" and masked the stench that drifted from mass graves. I do not think it is too much of a stretch to consider these people essential service providers: medical practitioners (men), herbal healers (women), clergy, and gravediggers.

Morbidity rates among this group were catastrophically high. Doctors, healers, and priests tended to the sick in plague houses (also called pesthouses), and gravediggers collected the bodies of those who had succumbed to the plague. By the second year of the plague, many cities, towns, and parishes in Europe were left without any of these people who either had died from the plague or fled when the horrors had become too much.

Fleeing Cities. Some people fled from the cities to the safety of the countryside. Here the populations were less dense and the chances of encountering plague-infected areas were thought to be less likely. The wealthy retired to secluded second residences; the poor simply fled, to fend and forage for themselves.

Responses to COVID-19

Now take a moment to reflect on the circumstances that we face presently. Which of Boccaccio's four categories of response are the closest to your own responses? Without much effort, I have updated Boccaccio's 14th-century descriptions to mirror our own circumstances.

Sheltering in Place. Those who have the resources to shelter in place spend time with their family, homeschooling children, chatting with friends online, eating and drinking (and trying to remain active so as not to put on the pounds), working, thinking, listening to music, playing with pets, streaming Netflix and Amazon Prime, venturing out to the grocery store for necessities, and abiding by social distancing rules.

Partying Like It Is the End of the World. Those students going on spring break vacations against CDC recommendations qualify for this category, as they reject social distancing. They are meeting up with strangers via dating apps, going to parks and beaches in large groups, and throwing parties in apartments without concern that they, even though asymptomatic, can spread the virus.

Going to Work to Provide Essential Services. (Thank you from the bottom of my heart!) This response includes all those working to keep our water running, electricity humming, Internet functional, garbage collected, sick treated and cared for, souls attended, supply chains running, drive-throughs open, packages delivered, fires extinguished, and streets safe. If I left your essential industry off this list, please accept my apologies.

Fleeing to the Countryside and Mountains. Stories from around the country and world have highlighted those who have fled to second homes. This response includes those who have enough extra income to flee urban hot spots and move to rural and small towns. (People in these less-populated areas would normally welcome visitors, but at the moment, they would rather see city dwellers remain in their own cities for fear of spreading COVID-19, a plausible concern.)

I urge you to think about the ways people reacted to the Black Death and compare those reactions with your own. What you may find is that our reactions to pandemics have not changed as much as we might think. What has changed is this: Doctors, nurses, and support staff from around the world are working on the front lines and in large research laboratories to beat this virus. History has shown us that they will succeed. But they need time. So until COVID-19 is driven back, be patient, be kind, be loving, and for heaven's sake—don't overindulge in partying!

William Landon is a professor of history who earned his PhD from the University of Edinburgh in the United Kingdom. He trusts that we can draw on history to understand our present circumstances because, despite our many contemporary advancements in technology, when we read other histories of pandemics we can always recognize ourselves in them. Landon has spent his entire career studying and writing about human history (our actions and motivations). He has delivered popular lectures and conference presentations on Renaissance Italy to audiences in the United States, Canada, Italy, England, Scotland, Germany, and Taiwan.

Know How Your Information Is Being Shared

Kevin Kirby

Informatics

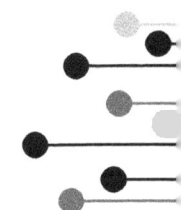

Informatics consists of a group of disciplines that deals with how humans engage with information. As such, informatics is about how we uncover and share information (journalism) and hide and protect it (cybersecurity). It is about processing information (computer science) and pulling insights out of raw data (statistics and data science). Informatics is about how information is communicated between people (interpersonal communication), across organizations (organizational communication) and strategically shaped for public consumption (public relations). It is about how businesses and governments can best put software to use (information systems) and build the digital tools we use to stay close (information technology). Informatics is even about how information stored in genes and proteins can be understood and manipulated (bioinformatics).[1]

In a time of crisis, information surges. We see daily reports on the spread of a virus conveyed in numbers, charts, maps, and animations. Investigative journalists expose hidden stories of tragedy and courage. Bystanders capture injustice by pointing their phone cameras, tapping a button, and sharing around the world. We are "together apart" as we use countless forms of media and technology to keep in touch. Yet just as informatics can help us stay safe and help us connect, it can also endanger us and set us against one another. The positive and negative aspects of informatics are inseparable.

In this idea paper, we will focus on *your* information. How informatics makes use of your information is becoming more and more important as we move deeper into the 21st century. And the COVID-19 pandemic in particular has brought an even tighter focus on the tension between sharing and hiding information, between what we as individuals want to keep private and what we want to make public. It also forces us to think of exactly who is consuming our information, and to what end.

Perhaps the most notable example is the flood of COVID-19 contact-tracing apps already on the market or being developed. These programs identify the places and moments when you may have come into contact with an infected person and then identify who you have come into contact with since. Massachusetts Institute of Technology (MIT) has made it a mission to monitor them and make their existence public. MIT has created a database of technology firms and technologists in a race to build apps that identify and notify people when they come into contact with a known (or perhaps suspected) carrier. A few of the app names are Stopp Corona, BeAware, and COVIDSafe. Depending on the country, some apps are more invasive than others in that they match up data including "citizens' identity, location, and even online payment history so that local police can watch for those who break quarantine rules."[2] Unless people are forced by a government or corporation to use an app, its effectiveness depends on people buying-in, or willingly entering their COVID-19 test results, and allowing the app to have access to their location at all times. If someone learns they have tested positive, they must agree to release a list of people they have been in contact with over the previous 14 days so those people can be notified.[3]

Suppose your employer asks you to download and install a mobile app that will help the company do contact tracing. The goal is to control the disease's transmission by interrupting its spread. Since it is all about uncovering and sharing information, contact tracing is a good example of the application of informatics. (Indeed, there is a field called health informatics.) It all sounds worthwhile. You try to be a good employee, and you download the app. It asks you to enable something called Location Services. You know this means someone can find you on a map. But who? It also wants to access your Bluetooth. The same technology that allows you to use wireless earbuds will also report on how close you are to others running this same app. You know it is building a list of your contacts. Do you want that? Your employer has purchased and probably customized the app, and even they may not be completely sure what the company that sold them the app will do with the data. In fact, you may find that you have multiple contact-tracing apps on your phone. Depending on the country in which you live, your government may have required you to install such an app on your phone (and you may be liable to prosecution if you leave home without it!).

We like to think we are the custodians, the caretakers, the *owners* of our information. We have all been warned to think carefully about what we share on social media, for example, because "the Internet never forgets." It is a responsibility most of us have come to accept or ignore at our own peril. Yet for every highly curated stream of social media posts that shapes our online identities, a hidden stream of information about us seeps out into the Internet. We may be vaguely aware of this, but it is easy to ignore.

Your degree of unease at using a contact-tracing app may vary. You might say, "It's just one app." There are countless archives of data about us from so many different sources. The online maps we use to guide us to a destination track our location and travel patterns using GPS technology. We leave a trail on the Internet as we visit websites. Our credit card transactions are stored. Swiping a loyalty card at a retailer profiles us by our purchases. Artificial intelligence has led to extremely powerful facial recognition, and it is becoming harder to avoid cameras in public. And then there is the rampant social media use: not just our posts but our likes, our retweets, and all the photos and references to us in the posts of our friends and followers.

In addition to the sheer number of sources of information about us, we must also confront the fact that this contact-tracing information can be even more revealing when combined by data aggregators. These are companies whose business is to use powerful algorithms to merge and process your multiple streams of information to produce new insights about you. Some databases that store anonymous information can be cleverly processed with other databases to reveal personally identifying information. The aggregators package and sell this data to other companies. That means it is never just about one app, like your employer's contact-tracing app. It is about that app's information about you *merged with everything else*. The collective value of the aggregated information about us is literally more valuable (to information buyers) than the sum of its parts because it tells a coherent story about you.

A well-known maxim attributed by the ancient Greek philosopher Plato to his teacher Socrates is "Know thyself." But if our self is made up of thousands of trillions of bytes of information scattered across the Internet and harvested by governments and companies, what does this mean? It is true that many of the large companies that store our information will show it to us upon request (Google and Facebook, for example). Yet the processing of this accessible information with information from other sources puts out of our reach the possibility of getting any global sense of what is known about us.

Because of this impracticality, a call to action such as *Know Your Information* is naïve. Knowing all the information about us is far beyond our capacity. However, there is a more practical call to action: *Know How Your Information Is Being Shared*. This means you must consider the interests of the people and organizations seeking your information. It means looking into the technologies behind the apps that share your information. It means studying the science of information protection (such as cryptology) and the capabilities of artificial intelligence. Do not be afraid to learn to write a little code! To rework another notable remark of Socrates: The unexamined app is not worth using.

In the end, a human-centered perspective is the most important. Informatics is often confused with one of its narrower subdisciplines, information technology. This misconception is natural, as we are surrounded by "tech." Yet as we have seen, tech is never just about tech. We can think of ourselves as merely *users* of technology, but this is not an acceptable fate in a crisis-ridden world. We need to take steps to become more knowledgeable and more skilled across the various disciplines that make up informatics, no matter what career or life path we choose. By taking these steps, we become savvier and more resilient against the forces of the aggregators. We become information creators, not just users, and a creator is in a much better position to face down crises, foreseen and unforeseen.

Kevin Kirby is dean of the College of Informatics and Evan and Lindsey Stein Professor of Biocomputing at Northern Kentucky University. After studying linguistics and mathematics, he earned his PhD in computer science from Wayne State University in his hometown of Detroit. His trust in the recommendation to know how your information is shared is grounded in his teaching and research in machine learning and artificial intelligence. He knows that confidentiality and privacy are difficult to preserve when computer systems allow personal records and interpersonal transactions to be shared so easily.

Turn to Mathematics to Know How We Are Doing

Phil McCartney

Mathematics

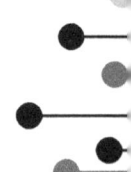

I recently learned that sociologists are guided by the motto "Things are not what they seem," which prompts them to not take things at face value but to look below the surface. It occurred to me that mathematicians and sociologists have more in common than one might guess. On the surface it may seem that mathematics is simply a quantitative discipline that crunches numbers using equations and algorithms. But mathematics is really about thinking through complex questions for which answers are not readily knowable. Obtaining answers to such purposeful questions may require persistence.

During times of crisis, those of us who have spent our careers teaching, learning, and doing mathematics likely have reflected on what habits of the mind our students can bring to decision making. Foremost among them is the ability to carry out a *thought experiment*, a problem-solving technique that involves finding solutions to complex questions and pressing issues.[1] These thought experiments are mentally rigorous exercises that apply mathematical principles to real-life challenges that have no easy answers. In fact, there may be more than one right answer (or there may be none). Students learn that making mathematical calculations with the aim of solving a problem takes considerable time and effort. To address the problem, they must work to find the best data they can, knowing that sometimes the data they would like to have does not exist.

The first step in conducting a thought experiment is asking a highly purposeful question. This first question launches the experiment and is referred to as asking "the right question" because of its critical role. You know when a question is right because it propels thought forward by triggering a series of additional questions to be answered, all of which clarify a path to solving the problem. The ability to ask such questions is one of the most important skills anyone can acquire. Some questions may lead to a dead end (this is actually helpful because now you know which path *not* to follow). Other questions move you along toward finding crucial insights.

Consider a thought experiment that addresses something on the mind of many people in the context of the COVID-19 pandemic. For illustrative purposes, a "right question" could be

> What, if any, are the health benefits of social distancing?[2] (If there are health benefits, can they be quantified?)

A multidisciplinary team of scientists, which included mathematicians, actually tackled this question when it examined social distancing interventions in six countries (China, South Korea, Italy, Iran, France, and the United States).[3] At the end of its research, the team estimated that the social distancing interventions imposed from January (when the virus emerged) to April 6, 2020, prevented or delayed 62 million COVID-19 cases that would have spread across the populations, resulting in an estimated 530 million infections in six countries.

The researchers did not simply come up with these numbers. They had to ask a series of right questions (with much discussion before attempting to answer them) to make these calculations. Below is the imagined thought process of the researchers and some of their questions and answers:

Q: What do we mean exactly by social distancing?

A: To answer this question, we identified a number of social distancing measures, including closure of schools, universities, and nonessential businesses; air travel restrictions; cancellation of large gatherings; and quarantining those people with infections or who had been exposed to infectious people. We also identified additional mandates, such as wearing masks; maintaining six feet of distance; prohibiting visitors to hospitals and nursing homes; paid sick leave; and declaring a state of emergency.

Q: What do social distancing mandates aim to change?

A: They aim to reduce the frequency of interaction between people so there are fewer opportunities to spread the virus that causes COVID-19.

Q: Now that we have a list of social distancing actions, how can we consolidate them into manageable categories?

A: We will categorize the social distancing measures into four main categories: (1) restricting travel, (2) cancellation of events and suspension of educational/commercial/religious activities, (3) quarantine, and (4) other policies.[4]

Q: What do we mean by health benefits?

A: For the purposes of this study, we will define the health benefits in terms of the lives saved from COVID-19-related deaths, illnesses avoided, and a reduction in people testing positive.

Q: How do we quantify social distancing mandates?

A: First, we need to find localities (e.g., in the United States, these might be found at the county level) that document the social distancing mandates issued. From this information, we can create a database. We need to ensure that this process is possible and then complete this step before we can move forward. It will not be easy to create this data set because we need to gather data from hundreds of sources in many languages. (In the end, the research team was able to compile a database consisting of 1,717 local, regional, and national documented mandates across the six countries.)

Q: Once we find localities with social distancing mandates, how do we determine compliance of these orders?

A: The reality is that not everyone will comply with any given mandate. Therefore, we have to make assumptions about the percentage of people who comply, but there must be a rationale for every assumption. We can base the percentage on the answers people give in surveys about the degree to which they are complying when they show COVID-19-like symptoms. (The researchers assumed that 70% of households with a symptomatic person had complied with the quarantine policy).

Q: How do we estimate the lives saved, illnesses avoided, and reduction in positive tests?

A: We can use the known rates by which people were dying, becoming ill, and testing positive and assume these rates would continue increasing for each locality in the absence of any social distancing measures, such as school closures and work-at-home mandates. (The research team compared actual rates for lives saved, illnesses avoided, and positive test cases reduced in each locality before social distancing was mandated and after each mandate had ended. Then they calculated "what-if" rates. That is, if social distancing mandates had not been put in place, by how much would the rates have increased?[5] To figure the numbers of lives saved, illnesses avoided, and cases reduced as indicated by positive tests, the researchers calculated the actual rates during distancing and the what-if rates. And those differences in the sets of rates allowed them to estimate how much each type of policy had contributed to flattening the curve.)

This Q&A series covers only some of the questions the research team might have asked and answered in their thought experiment. Implementing the Q&A process was absolutely critical because it promoted direct deep thinking and allowed the team to move forward, step by step, to solve an extremely challenging problem.

As you can see, thought experiments are important for estimating the effects of actions taken, such as the role of social distancing in the spread of COVID-19. During this pandemic, mathematical principles (e.g., modeling) have been used to address other critical questions. One such question is, at what point might infections drop to a rate of one case per 1 million people?

That is the rate at which some medical experts believe social distancing mandates can end. Thought experiments allow us to consider these what-if scenarios and then predict what might happen. They are powerful tools to grasp situations that at first might appear beyond understanding.

Thought experiments spark students to develop habits of the mind that will serve them well for their entire lives. The world would benefit greatly if our students were to engage in such thought. But the experience of using deep mathematical thinking should not be limited to individuals with access to elite academic programs. The public interest is best served when challenging educational opportunities are broadly available. In fact, the world we live in demands a well-educated public—a public that insists on accuracy and transparency in data and how that data is used to make the models that drive policy decisions.

Phil McCartney is an associate professor of mathematics who earned his PhD from Claremont Graduate University. He trusts in the power of mathematics to discover truth and to foster good decision-making. Math relies on the integrity of the data gatherers because the math itself is only as good as the quality of the data that is put into its equations. Our government, corporations, and other entities that want answers should invest in gathering quality data.

Support the Artists You Turn to in Times of Crisis

Jason Vest

Music

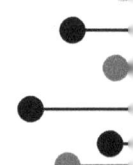

The discipline of music is a large area of study within the performing arts in which artistic expression is traditionally conveyed to a live audience through the voice, the body, and sounds generated through instruments or other objects. Music itself can be defined as alternations of sound over time to make what we might call a rhythm and/or a melody. For as long as humans have recorded history, music has been used as a social tool to communicate messages, meaning, and values.

Music long preceded speech as a form of human communication and thus is deeply rooted in our physiology.[1] It is a powerful cultural tool that can unite people and transcend differences. Music is interwoven with our identity and sense of what it means to be human. People also use music as a form of escapism when they want to relax and take a break from life's challenges. Scientific findings demonstrate music's ability to ameliorate mood, anxiety, fear, depression, and overall health.[2]

The COVID-19 pandemic altered lives and routines throughout the world. Work schedules were interrupted, lives lost, and fear and anxiety heightened. During times of uncertainty, people reach out for music and other entertainment as we deal with difficult emotions and adjust to a very different everyday routine. This coronavirus pandemic has given many people more time at home during the day—time we used to spend commuting or going to the gym. More than ever, people are turning to and sharing music for entertainment, healing, and comfort.

Musicians who depend on their craft for income have responded to the pandemic in remarkable ways. Even without work and money coming in, some artists have continued to create music and communicate hope and healing through livestream shows, often recorded from the musicians' homes. Other videos feature artists singing and playing instruments from front steps or balconies, all while facing the prospect that their livelihood may vanish for a year or more.

The Science of Music

Music has been marginalized in the United States as merely entertainment, a distraction from the travails of hard work. Our education systems view music as ancillary to reading and math, which is reflected in budget cuts to the arts programs in public schools. But music is known to be extremely beneficial to learning. Studies repeatedly show that reading and math scores improve when students are exposed to musical experiences or when music is part of their school curriculum. These studies are important because they demonstrate that music helps us become better learners and workers. Still, the general public fails to recognize how essential music is to our well-being and health.

Given our species' long history with music, it is not surprising to hear of its positive effects on our minds and bodies. Music acts as a kind of therapy because listening to or playing it releases neurochemical and hormonal agents, activating metabolic processes, regulating mind and body.[3] Music reaches into the deeper structures of the brain (the limbic system), where emotions and memory interact to regulate the endocrine and autonomic nervous systems. Thus, while music can evoke emotion solely through a melody or rhythm, it can also have a profound effect on our mental and physical well-being.[4]

Music and Trauma

The COVID-19 pandemic has caused trauma for many, experienced as deep grief and emotional turmoil. The families of those who have died have suffered a pain often exacerbated by not being with the ailing in their final days. Tens of millions have lost their jobs, with no certainty about if or when they will return to work. Businesses, investments, and retirement funds have been diminished by an unpredictable stock market. Meanwhile, news headlines, social media posts, and conversations are dominated by a virus that has upended our way of life and injected fear into the most mundane of tasks, such as grocery shopping or pumping gas.

Most of us can recall important moments in our lives when music calmed feelings or helped make sense of grief and pain. For instance, it is rare to attend a funeral and not hear music of some kind. Traumatic events are often accompanied by memories of the music that helped us heal or that reminds us of a loved one. Music helps us process our grief and express our feelings.

The use of creative arts in trauma therapy has gained wide acceptance because of the ability of the arts to give expression to trauma that has yet to be processed into a narrative or expressed verbally. Specifically, music is associated with the right hemisphere of the brain and the limbic system, which hold memories and emotions that are often unprocessed. The left hemisphere of the brain deals more with the verbal and rational and often has great difficulty forming a coherent narrative for trauma. Music and other creative art therapies allow emotions to surface slowly, giving the left brain the time and ability to process trauma and grief into a narrative, thus allowing the subject to move toward acceptance.[5]

Our Obligation to Artists

Changes in listening patterns since the onset of the COVID-19 pandemic further show how music is a human response to grief. Spotify reports that listeners are consuming less "danceable" music and focusing on more "chill," mood-oriented music with calmer tempos and lower energy.[6] Pandora has seen increased streaming in the categories "Wind-Down," "Focus," and "Family." Deezer has seen playlists like "Cozy Coffeeshop" jump by 486% and "Mellow Days" by 305%.[7] On-demand music videos have also increased.[8] However, with the exception of country music and children's music, overall online streaming has declined and physical sales are down by one third. On the other hand, direct-to-fan performances, at no cost to viewers and usually conducted from the artists' homes, have increased.[9]

During quarantine, some live online musical performances have soared.[10] Classical musicians have gained much wider engagement than before COVID-19. Instagram introduced Verzuz Battles, where two established artists go head-to-head (Erykah Badu vs. Jill Scott were in a live performance where fans voted for a winner). Yo-Yo Ma has posted solo performances during quarantine using the hashtag #SongsOfComfort, with many performances receiving up to a million views. Musicians of all genres have reached out and shared music, often with no expectation of remuneration. This has been especially remarkable among artists such as classical musicians whose entire income depends on live performances in front of an audience.

Why would these artists continue to create music for consumption without any monetary reward? At the core, musicians are communicators and create art to connect. They train for decades to cultivate their talent so they can better communicate the ideas and feelings that flow from music. Musicians are collaborative; without other musicians and an audience, both their income and sense of purpose are removed. Also, by continuing to perform and connect with their audience, musicians avoid disconnecting from their fans and others in the music community.

While musicians are not being paid to perform live, organizations and entertainment companies profit from the exposure that these performances bring at a time when people have free time and crave escapism. The Metropolitan Opera, the Vienna State Opera, and others offer free streaming of past performances, which has been extremely successful. At the same time, many of these organizations have laid off all their workers for the foreseeable future. Concert tours have been cancelled, impacting not only the musicians but the behind-the-scenes support professionals who make the money-making performances happen. Professional choristers and soloists have suddenly had all engagements cancelled indefinitely, with no assurance of performances happening in the future. By one estimate, 45.5% of jobs within the category "performing arts and spectator sports" were lost between February and April 2020 as theaters, concert halls, and dance companies closed.[11] And many musicians in the U.S. economy are gig workers and independent contractors.

We should recognize that the musicians who reach out to help us heal and work through our grief are in tenuous positions. Even as they, too, are suffering, artists continue to make music so that others will be comforted and not feel alone. Our society must value musicians and music, if only because of the powerful effects music has on our mental and physical health.

Our support of musicians must go beyond attending an occasional concert and offering verbal encouragement. Whenever you have an opportunity to access music for free, remember that it is not actually free. Think about what you gain from the music you are listening to, then pay it forward in support of the larger music community.

How do you pay it forward? Listen to their livestreams (and donate to the organizations they fundraise for), help strengthen music-focused non-profits such as the National Endowment for the Arts, support arts funding in the schools, and advocate for musicians to receive a living wage. When you do this, remember the science that tells us music has a profound effect on our well-being and plays a central role in helping us cope with trauma and grieve for our loss.

Jason Vest earned his doctorate in vocal music performance from the University of Kentucky. He has also earned an MBA. He is a university administrator, professor of voice, and performer, who rehearses or performs about 10 to 14 days of every month, often traveling throughout the United States and Europe. The COVID-19 pandemic and the subsequent cancellations of performances have affected his family's income for the near future, but he is fortunate among performers to have a full-time job that he can lean on. Vest's colleagues who perform full-time have suddenly seen their life's training and work come to a halt and have no idea when or if "normal" will ever return. He trusts in the body of scientific evidence that verifies music's healing power and its effects on personal and societal well-being. As further support to music's power, it has been a part of human life since the beginning of recorded history.

Understand That Crises Can Be Managed

Nana Arthur-Mensah

Organizational Leadership

Organizational leadership is a field of study that focuses on what it means to be an effective leader in a variety of settings. It seeks to develop the skills and knowledge to manage people, relationships, and resources in order to achieve organizational goals. Students of organizational leadership learn to negotiate and implement change, work with diverse groups in global and local settings, and engender positive and productive working environments. In organizational leadership (OL) programs, students study individual and team dynamics, assess their own leadership style and skills, and wrestle with ethical dilemmas.

In times of crisis such as COVID-19, we turn to local, national, and global leaders for answers and guidance, even as they themselves are trying to navigate and adapt to turbulent times. Particularly in this pandemic, we look to those who provide guidance and hope and who inspire the best choices for ourselves, our families, and our communities. These leaders could be CEO's, mentors, counselors, activists, governors, doctors, or spiritual teachers, among others.

It is safe to say that none of our students, faculty, or staff have ever before experienced a global pandemic that threatens livelihoods, economies, and organizations. In fact, one can argue that no leader could have fully prepared for COVID-19's large-scale ramifications. Regardless, effective leaders understand that crises have three phases—pre-crisis, crisis, and post-crisis—and each requires a different skill set to navigate it successfully.[1]

In the pre-crisis phase, leaders anticipate crises by moving their organization from crisis-vulnerable to crisis-ready. They continuously scan the environment, looking to identify warnings or threats on the horizon that could cripple the organization and its ability to survive and thrive. This level of alertness and knowledge gathering helps the leader and team prepare for the threat. Strategies include securing the adequate resources to respond and making plans to allocate them where and when needed. An effective leader is always on the lookout for signs of an impending crisis. Leaders who read broadly and listen openly put themselves in a position to anticipate and prepare not for a specific crisis but for any crisis that would disrupt normal operations.

As a crisis unfolds, people look to their leaders. This is the time when a leader must guide behavior and actions. Leaders acknowledge and articulate the grave danger to the organization and its members, relying on their team members or trusted advisors for expert advice and support for decision-making and action-taking. In the crisis phase, the goal is to contain the fallout and to rally with others to find solutions, such as slowing or preventing the spread of the coronavirus and ensuring that people have resources for survival.

Understandably, leaders face stress and anxiety as they manage an increasingly fluid situation while trying to juggle needs and make sound decisions for organizations and their members. During times of high uncertainty, some fundamental questions swirl in the minds of leaders: What can the organization do to survive the crisis? What character traits and skills can I exhibit to build trust? How do I inspire and mobilize others to be part of the solutions? Who should I be looking to for informed recommendations? How can I stay abreast of where the greatest needs are?

Leaders must understand their own strengths and weaknesses and how their emotional responses impact others. When emotions are raw and millions of people are dealing with loss and insecurity, people look to leaders who exude confidence, calmness, and optimism, even when the situation is dire. Those are the leaders who exhibit the five pillars of emotional intelligence: self-awareness, self-regulation, motivation, empathy, and social skills. Leaders who demonstrate these qualities in the face of challenges can motivate others to act.

Because events unfold so quickly in a crisis, there is no time for misinformation. No matter how grim the situation, people want to know the truth. Clear and honest communication is key as leaders seek to understand and respond to needs and concerns. Leaders can gain trust even when the decisions they make may affect people negatively. There may be layoffs, a loss of services, closures, and pay cuts, but members will stand by leaders who are authentic and act in the best interest of the organization, such as balancing economics and public health.

In crisis, there are no blueprints, but theories of leadership offer a kind of road map for action. Adaptive, authentic, and transformational leadership are particularly instructive for the COVID-19 pandemic. Adaptive leaders establish a safe space where members can openly discuss their fears and hopes. In this safe space, people can explore their beliefs and assumptions about the organization, its leaders, and the situation. Leaders can also use this space to assure people they are valued, to negotiate conflicting perspectives, and to elicit feedback.

Authentic leaders do not deceive or intentionally misinform. The leader builds legitimacy through honest relationships that welcome input and openness. This style builds trust and support, which motivates individual and team performance. These leaders stand in contrast to those who emphasize profit and share price over the well-being of workers and the overall health of the organization and society.

Transformational leaders know that in times of change, people respond best when they are empowered. Such leaders are thoughtful and inclusive.

They inspire others to adapt, create a shared vision, and execute change. These leaders welcome contributions at all levels, challenging people to take ownership and surpass their perceived capabilities. They trust people to innovate and create to overcome difficulties and find solutions. Transformational leaders recognize the strengths of the people they are leading and know how to put those strengths to best use. But they also accept the weaknesses of their people.

In the post-crisis phase, the threat is contained and life returns to some semblance of normalcy. Leaders now have to grapple with the fallout and recovery. This is a time for retrospective sense making, a process that requires reviewing and analyzing what has transpired since the crisis began.[2] They must reflect on their level of preparedness and adaptability. Leaders have to ask tough questions about what was overlooked, neglected, or carelessly dismissed. Many leaders will learn that their organization neglected to invest in a learning and growth culture. While it is tempting to place blame during this period, leaders must identify the human biases, institutional failures, or special interest groups that were barriers to crisis prevention and adaptation.[3] This post-crisis phase also includes making significant structural changes to address the aftermath while inspiring personnel to adapt to a new reality.

In times of crisis, we encourage our students to observe effective and ineffective leaders around them. Some leaders display heroic and inspirational leadership, while others leave us shaking our heads in disbelief. Yet we can learn from both. When we understand the complexities of leadership, we can ask ourselves what kind of leader we want to be and know the work it takes to become that leader. If you are an emerging or current leader, know that becoming an effective leader does not occur overnight; much work is involved. Understand, too, that a crisis has phases, and each can be managed. Make it your obligation to learn how to anticipate and negotiate a crisis to build a better reality afterward.

Nana Arthur-Mensah is an assistant professor of organizational leadership. She earned her doctorate in educational leadership and organizational development from the University of Louisville. She trusts the idea that leaders can learn to manage crises because leadership is a developmental process. Leaders become successful and effective with experience and by taking steps to intentionally develop skills and knowledge. This is well documented in literature on leadership and also in countless biographies and autobiographies of leaders. Having lived and worked in Ghana, the United Kingdom, and the United States, Arthur-Mensah enjoys meeting new people and learning about other cultures, traveling, reading, and listening to music.

IDEA 19

Stand Up for the Marginalized and Vulnerable

Yaw A. Frimpong-Mansoh

Philosophy

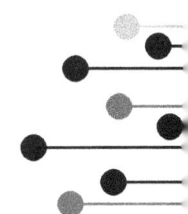

Philosophers work primarily through deep thinking and reasoning to ask questions about things such as the nature of existence, morality, and knowledge. Within the discipline of philosophy, the specialty of ethics is concerned with morals (ideas of right and wrong) and values that guide actions and decision making.

In the midst of the COVID-19 crisis, philosophers take interest in the ethics underlying the countless decisions that policy makers and citizens have made (or have to make) to address this pandemic. For example, the mandates and guidelines regarding social distancing, stay-at-home orders, and closures raise ethical questions about the values of individual liberty versus the common (public) good.

So how do people decide between individual liberty and the public good, especially in times of crisis? In siding with one value over the other, we must ask what counts as the public good. For example, is it better to protect hospitals from being overwhelmed or to protect the economy from collapsing? We must also consider whose liberties are sacrificed in the name of the public good. Should meatpacking workers risk their health to meet the needs of a meat-eating society and to keep the food chain moving?

Critical thinking and ethical reflection are required to answer such complex questions. Philosophy offers two major ethical frames (among others) to guide these answers: the utilitarian frame and the egalitarian frame.

Utilitarian Ethical Frame

A utilitarian ethical frame prompts a decision maker to think in terms of the greatest good for the most people. Decisions based on utilitarian principles allow the interests of some people to be sacrificed to serve the interests of the majority. Seventy-year-old Texas Lieutenant Governor Dan Patrick applied this principle during the COVID-19 pandemic when he weighed the health dangers to the elderly against the financial losses from not reopening the economy. Although he himself is in a high-risk age category, he was willing to risk the survival of his age group in exchange for keeping the economy open. In a television interview, Patrick contended, "There are more important things than living. And that's saving this country for my children and my grandchildren and saving this country for all of us."[1]

President Trump applied the utilitarian principle when he invoked the Defense Production Act ordering meatpacking plants to stay open. He made this decision because when plants close down, millions of pounds of meat are backlogged, which has cascading effects on the rest of the food chain. Farmers are affected because they have nowhere to send their pigs, cattle, and poultry, forcing them to consider euthanizing their livestock. The interruption of the food supply triggers panic buying, further exacerbating the problem. By keeping the meatpacking lines running, Trump sided with the greater good of the food supply chain over the health and safety of the workers. This order forced employees to work in crowded and highly contagious environments. To compound matters, the Occupational Safety and Health Administration (OSHA) did not enforce safety guidelines as long as the corporations showed good faith efforts to keep workers safe.

The utilitarian frame is a slippery slope to maximizing the interests (e.g., economic benefits) of the majority (typically the dominant groups) at the expense of racial and ethnic minority groups and other vulnerable peoples. The infamous Tuskegee Study conducted by the U.S. Public Health Service between 1932 and 1972 illustrates the danger of this approach. In that study, 600 impoverished African American sharecroppers—399 with syphilis, and 201 without—took part in a supposed clinical vaccine trial. However, the real purpose was for researchers to observe the natural course of the disease for better understanding. The researchers never informed the participants they had syphilis. Instead, the men were told their treatment was for "bad blood." For over 40 years, the men went untreated as the researchers monitored the disease's progression. Public health officials who oversaw this unethical research justified it on the grounds that they were serving the public good. But in doing this, they disregarded the dignity and humanity of that minority group.[2]

Egalitarian Ethical Frame

Egalitarian ethics is much more concerned with justice and equality. It is centered in treating people in a fair way. One form of the egalitarian ethical principle is the frame put forth by philosopher John Rawls as an antidote to the utilitarian method. Rather than highlighting the greater good, this approach emphasizes the needs of the most vulnerable.

Rawls's egalitarian frame draws on a metaphor called the "veil of ignorance." The veil of ignorance is a mental exercise that asks decision makers to imagine that they exist behind a veil of ignorance about themselves. (Know that *ignorance* here means "a lack of knowledge or information"; we are all ignorant about many things.) Behind this veil, a person imagines that they know nothing about themselves—their abilities, their individual tastes, or their status in society, including their identities such as gender, race, and country of origin.

Rawls saw this mental exercise as one path to a just society in which no one has an unfair advantage over others.[3] When we make decisions, we usually have plenty of information about ourselves but lack information (or are ignorant) about others. To remedy this, decision makers must take steps to be as objective and unbiased as possible, not letting their own interests influence public policies. This process requires "forgetting about" or "ignoring" the needs tied to the decision makers' own social identities and positions in society. In other words, decision makers must work hard to act as if they are ignorant of their own personal situations and self-interests.

If this exercise sounds challenging, it is. How many people can make decisions without considering how they (and people like themselves) will be affected? But by pretending they sit behind a veil of ignorance, they are more likely to be objective, fair, and adhere to what Rawls calls the *difference principle*. This principle maintains that decisions should benefit the least advantaged, because when the most vulnerable benefit, we all benefit. Under this principle, caring for vulnerable populations, such as the elderly, the incarcerated, the unhoused, and the uninsured, means caring for the nation as a whole. Rawls's call for fair decision-making is consistent with Dr. Martin Luther King's powerful statement: "Injustice anywhere is a threat to justice everywhere."

Rawls's egalitarian frame offers people a guide to assess the many responses made during the COVID-19 pandemic. It challenges us to help improve the well-being of the vulnerable and disadvantaged. Consider the vulnerability of African Americans across the United States who disproportionately test positive for and die from COVID-19. In Chicago, for example, African Americans, who make up 32% of the city's population, represent more than half of all positive COVID-19 test results and 72% of virus-related deaths. Dr. Anthony Fauci, the director of the National Institute of Allergy and Infectious Diseases, attributes the disparate impact to a structural problem in America. Fauci remarked that the coronavirus is "shining a bright light" on "unacceptable" health disparities for African Americans[4] and others.

National crises like the COVID-19 pandemic expose the vulnerability of our humanity: Each of us is a potentially vulnerable individual in need of support. Here we see a confirmation of the African Ubuntu philosophy, which defines the identity of our humanity: "I am because we are, and since we are I am."

Our humanity is interlinked, and we survive and thrive on the shoulders of one another, in mutual support. The call to action is to become humanitarians, not only in times of crisis. This call includes embracing the wisdom in a system of distributive justice, one that uplifts the vulnerable and the least advantaged in our communities.

Yaw A. Frimpong-Mansoh earned his PhD from the University of Alberta. He is a professor of philosophy and the director of the philosophy program at Northern Kentucky University. He trusts in deep thinking and reasoning because both require considering many different perspectives, without being reactive. Deep thinking also emphasizes thoroughly exploring and evaluating moral principles before applying them. Frimpong-Mansoh was born and raised in Ghana, in West Africa. He relocated with his family to the United States in 2002 and is an American citizen. His research is primarily in the areas of bioethics and health care ethics. He coauthored the book Bioethics in Africa: Theories and Praxis *(2019). He has also published articles in international journals.*

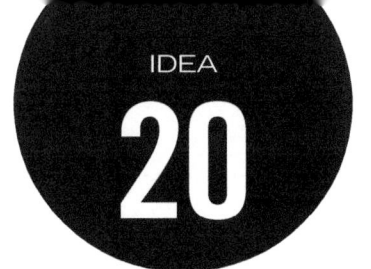

Join Together in an Age of Apart

Ryan Salzman

Political Science

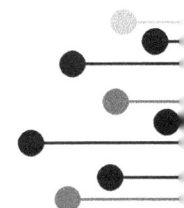

Political science is the study of politics, or the activities that relate to governance at all levels.[1] Those activities include the processes of government (e.g., how a bill becomes a law); the workings of the executive, legislative, and judicial branches of government; the behavior of those in government; and the ways people interact with governments. Political scientists view the distribution of political power as a puzzle. The pieces of the puzzle include individuals, groups, institutions, and the relative power each holds at any given moment.

Democracies are the messiest of all political systems, especially relative to, say, a dictatorship, where people do not have the power or right to influence decisions or actions. Democracies protect the rights of people to freely associate, speak their opinions, and engage in civic action. The democracy puzzle has the most pieces, and the least inherently powerful piece—"the people"—is most central to a democracy functioning well.

In the United States, a fundamental aspect of democracies is the central role played by associations—groups of individuals with a common interest, often under the support and protection of a formal organization. The people of a democracy display associational behaviors, such as forming and joining groups, which serve as both support and delimiters for political leadership.

In times of crisis, the puzzle pieces can be totally reconfigured. For example, the COVID-19 pandemic has elevated the role of political leadership in making highly nuanced decisions around which jobs are considered essential or nonessential, how resources are acquired and distributed to address COVID-19, and what timelines are appropriate for instituting and ending social distancing mandates.

Social distancing rules constrain the people's abilities to associate with one another. To control the spread of the virus, people have been asked to stay at home, avoid group activities, and limit contact with those outside of their households. Under the shadow of the pandemic, associating with our friends, family, and neighbors has been markedly different. But without the structure of associations, U.S. democracy is in real trouble.[2] This is a time when the people must adapt and innovate to find new ways to associate.

Associating Pre-COVID-19

Before the pandemic, people responded to issues that mattered to them by gathering face-to-face, working together, and rallying in each other's presence to overcome issues confronting our country. Without the ability of individuals to band together, communicate, debate, and advocate regularly, it is doubtful democratic governance can work effectively.[3] It is nearly impossible for individual Americans of modest means to pressure elected and agency officials in a large, republican-style democracy.

Whether we know it or not, every aspect of human life is, or can become, political. There is probably no aspect of life that is ungoverned by some law or regulation.[4] That is why decision-making cannot be left in the hands of a few but must be within reach of us all. Associational behavior allows people with similar needs and interests to join together in groups (e.g., neighborhood watch groups, theater groups, parent-teacher groups, and Planned Parenthood and abortion alternative centers).[5] Connecting the individual to others is the foundation of our democratic system. Because associations serve a bridging function, they bestow a social capital (the power of connections or the group) on its members and the organization. Social capital is important for political activity, because people and associations can draw on that capital when they are compelled to act. The more this kind of social capital exists, the stronger the democracy is.[6]

The Importance of Associating During a Pandemic

Because people have been severely constrained by social distancing mandates, strategies to support associations need immediate attention. Traditional ways of associating are on pause. Recreational leagues, gardening associations, and book clubs, all premised on convening in person, have either gone virtual or been put on hold. While people focus their attention on the crisis at hand, associations are not their most immediate concern; therefore, the tools of assembly are compromised. Democratic power is weakened because the people cannot be easily mobilized to oppose the actions of political elites.

In a world where social distancing persists, elite-centered interest groups benefit greatly. Powerful and well-funded interest groups, such as banking, oil, and pharmaceutical lobbies, have not missed a step during the COVID-19 crisis. For the most part, lobbyists need not worry about a congressperson's constituents flooding their office or holding public rallies to fight specific policies. Professional lobbyists for major corporations and other well-funded interest groups continue to be well paid. To be clear, some lobbyists do advocate for policies that benefit the people, but they are a minority, and those lobbyists often rely on mobilizing citizen groups to maintain balance with corporate lobbyists.

Strategic associational behavior is needed now more than ever to ensure the constitution of our society and to balance interests in politics. Though associating online is not new, it has reached a level of importance unimaginable just a few months ago. It is possible for us to network, establish and grow feelings of mutual trust, and advocate for policy change from our computers.

But online associations cannot compete with the strength of face-to-face interactions for building social capital or confronting professional lobbyists. Although social distancing is important, the importance of in-person interactions cannot be underestimated. Conversations before, after, and during meetings enhance social capital and often lead to further interactions, strengthening societal bonds and empowering individuals and ideas in the democratic framework. In a democracy, there is only one way forward: together.

We can be called to physically gather, even during the COVID-19 pandemic. Such an example can be found in the Black Lives Matter (BLM) movement, where the rules on congregating were suspended by the force of a moral shock.[7] In this case, the moral shock happened with watching a white police officer kneel on George Floyd's neck for almost nine minutes, resulting in a visceral unease among the people. This brazen act elicited such a response that it united diverse peoples behind the BLM movement, compelling them to join demonstrations aimed at abolishing, defunding, or changing the policing system. Unable to stay silent, tens of thousands of Americans left their homes and marched in one of the most far-reaching mass protests in U.S. history.[8,9]

But the occurrence of protests during the crisis does not mean that people should organize and gather the same as before the pandemic. In a world without physical gathering, the force of traditional associations must be reestablished, even if the means of associating are nontraditional. And if physical protests and other mass assemblies are necessary (as with the BLM protests), we should employ the strategies outlined below.

Make Virtual Meetings as Effective as In-Person Meetings. Learn the features of virtual meeting software and teach it to others for more effective and productive facilitation and interaction. For instance, using the small-group breakout sessions feature can make meetings feel more natural and similar to in-person meetings.

Create More Groups. We need to meet more, even if only online. Start a virtual book club or happy hour. Host a video chat for kids. Create subcommittees for special projects that traditional groups can focus on during the crisis. The content of meetings—business, leisure, civics—is less important than the act of connecting with one another. There is no such thing as too many groups.

Replace "Politics" With "Civics." Although people tend to avoid talking "politics," they are usually more open to "civics"—actions we can take as citizens in our communities. Creating virtual groups around local civic concerns can be important for the issues they address *and* the potential of that group to (eventually) talk politics beyond the local level.

Make a Demonstration. People can do many things locally to influence policies in their community, even while social distancing practices are in place. Those actions, maximized by social media sharing of compelling content, can inspire group conversations. Products of demonstration are public art, Little Free Libraries, community gardening, and temporary pedestrian and bicycle infrastructure.[10] Investing valuable resources in these types of civic projects sends a message to policy makers about what is important to the people. Sharing these actions online invites interaction and virtual engagement, which further demonstrates their importance to policy makers.

Practice Social Distancing When Attending Demonstrations. When you attend a protest or demonstration, wear a mask, do not touch others, sanitize your hands frequently, and self-quarantine afterward.

Think Local. Take time to learn about the important policies that are shaped primarily at the local level, and make those your focus. You may find that you have been overlooking the most important political venue for realizing your personal political goals. Local engagement is doable under any circumstance, and it is excellent practice for further engagement at higher levels of government. Also, it is less difficult to initiate associational behaviors around local politics because they are less partisan, and your friends and neighbors have a vested interest.

Now is the time to commit to associational behavior, even if social distancing is still necessary. Remember that in a democratic system, forming and joining groups is fundamental. Democracies give us the rights to freely associate, express our opinions, and engage in political action. Do not take those rights for granted.

Ryan Salzman is an associate professor of political science. He earned his PhD in political science from the University of North Texas. He trusts the importance of associations as the cornerstone of democracy because they are the path for ordinary people to gain political power. Associations change, but people associating is constant. As an educator, researcher, elected official, and community activist, Salzman has witnessed the power of people associating to affect political outcomes. Modern democracy has worked this way for over 200 years, and there is no reason to think it will change even under these novel conditions.

Imagine How the Pandemic Affects Everyone Across the Lifespan

Allyson S. Graf

Psychological Science

Psychology is the scientific study of the mind and behavior. One area within psychology is lifespan development, which examines the ways human beings change as we age and move through each life stage (e.g., infancy, adolescence, middle adulthood, and so on) in similar yet unique ways. Lifespan psychologists consider the full human life cycle, beginning with conception and ending with death. At any given moment in the life cycle, we are a product of the timing of our birth in history, the years we have lived, and our present-day experiences.[1]

Here I draw attention to the complexity of human development to illustrate how the COVID-19 outbreak, or any significant event, impacts people and elicits different responses, depending on age; creates a "coming-of-age" story for some cohorts; and alters the path of everyone's life. Below are six principles that serve as a framework for assessing these dynamics. While not exhaustive, taken together they give us reason to show understanding, empathy, and compassion for ourselves and for those in other stages of the lifespan.

No Matter Our Place in the Lifespan, We Are Always Responding to Change

Everyone experiences age-related changes that are both maturational (e.g., puberty) and social in nature (e.g., expected age to retire).[2] These experiences are further complicated by their gender, race/ethnicity, sexual orientation, disability status, and other social statuses and identifiers. People are constantly responding to change, although the impetus behind the change is not usually as dramatic and widespread as what we have seen with this virus. Regardless of age, COVID-19 has changed the course of everyone's life, albeit in different ways.

Our experiences with, and our responses to, the pandemic are shaped by our physical status and our capabilities for understanding the world. Clearly, how we respond to the challenges the pandemic brings depends on where we are in the lifespan. People who have been in the workforce for 20 years and lost their job as a result of COVID-19 may be preoccupied with how to pay household bills. A 16-year-old who lost a first job may brush it off as no big deal. A young adult may struggle with finding love during lockdown. All these concerns are developmentally typical. [3,4]

People Are Capable of Change, Even in a Crisis

Humans are capable of adapting in times of change, even if it becomes more challenging as we age. Adapting draws on effort, time, money, and energy. Where we are in the lifespan affects the types of resources we have at our disposal which in turn affects how we respond. COVID-19 has altered everyone's routines.[5] School, work, leisure, and other areas of life have changed drastically. Such disruptions have created cascading concerns about well-being, the future, and whether things will return to normal.

The ability to pivot in times of crisis and harness one's resources underlies the psychological concept of resiliency, a person's capacity to recover from difficulties. That capacity is bolstered by previous experiences with challenging circumstances from which they recovered and grew. The capacity to be resilient is compromised when experiences leave a person feeling defeated and unable to recover. Resiliency can be learned, and a key lesson is that there are multiple pathways to personal fulfillment. For example, people working in the performing arts who lose their jobs during the pandemic exhibit resiliency when they can identify future opportunities, such as offering private lessons through Zoom, returning to school, looking into a backup career, or using time to work on a craft (songwriting, recording, painting).

Human Development Is Multidimensional

The way people grow and change across the lifespan has many interrelated dimensions—biological (or physical), cognitive, and social—each of which has subcomponents. For example, the cognitive dimension involves, among other things, thinking, remembering, and perceiving. But what we think and remember is intertwined with our brain maturation and social experiences. Whether or not we contract COVID-19 depends on interacting factors. For example, the strength of our immune system (biological), how we perceive the virus (cognitive), and who we live with (social) all combine to increase or decrease our chance of becoming infected.

Regarding the biological dimension, as children are developing, they are building their immune system function; as people move toward old age, the immune system function declines, making older adults more susceptible to infection with and complications of COVID-19. Cognitively, a

5-year-old may perceive the virus as a monster, and an 80-year-old may perceive the virus as something they cannot fight off like when they were younger. Regarding the social aspect, children tend to live in households with parents or guardians and other siblings. Adults in old age are more likely to live alone, with one other person, or be at higher risk in congregate settings.

Change Involves Losses but Also Gains

When we assess any change to our lives, we must consider not only what we have lost but also what we have gained. If loss is the focus, we are unaware of the possible good that can come out of change. If our graduation ceremony was cancelled, that is a loss. But we gained from the love and care of people who arranged new kinds of celebrations. When we lost our routines to COVID-19, many of us found ourselves with more time on our hands. But perhaps we finally took the time to learn a technology that once seemed too complicated. Or maybe we chose to spend more time appreciating nature. The ability to recognize that hope can be found in dark times is the antidote to being overwhelmed by loss and opens opportunities for growth and connection to others. We must look for positives, no matter how small.

Human Development Is Contextual

Your experience is unique to the particular place and time you were born. So, your 80-year old neighbor is experiencing this pandemic differently than a 25-year-old college student. People in Kentucky are experiencing COVID-19 differently than people in Florida. People in large cities do not have the same experience as those in rural areas. "Experiencing differently" also encompasses a multitude of settings—home, local neighborhood, school or work, healthcare, place of worship—and spans multiple layers of influence— physical, psychological, relational, financial, spiritual, and so on. We cannot fathom the magnitude of ways in which people are experiencing COVID-19. Your experiences cannot be the same as mine, but whatever they are, they are shaping our development.

We also need a nod here to the historical context. COVID-19 occurred in a time of history when digital technologies dominate. So, we have to sort through a 24-hour news cycle, the countless news sources, and instant sharing of information. That did not exist in the influenza pandemic of 1918 when information spread slowly and from few sources. Peoples' pandemic experiences in 1918 were very different from today. That, however, does not mean we can't find similarities. At both times, people wrestled with what information to believe. They also had to find ways to avoid contracting the virus while still connecting with others.

Coming-of-Age Events Define a Generation

Large-scale historical events, such as the Great Depression and September 11, affect everyone who is alive at the time. But we also think of these events as defining the generation that happens to be "coming of age" then.[6] Baby boomers (those born between 1946 and 1963) came of age after World War II, a prosperous time for the United States, and were strongly impacted by the Cold War's nuclear arms race. They were also shaped by the Vietnam War and the assassinations of Dr. Martin Luther King Jr. and John F. Kennedy. As a result, their fears are grounded in a clearly defined entity (e.g., a nuclear arms race and the Soviet Union challenging U.S. lives and values). Further, these coming-of-age events have influenced the perceptions of every other event that baby boomers have experienced since.

Generation Z (those born between 1996 and 2015) grew up in the aftermath of 9/11 and live in a world where gun violence and terrorism are defined as the threats. In other words, their fears are centered around individuals or small numbers of people infiltrating public spaces (church, school, airplane, mall), intent on carrying out violence, mayhem, and death that reverberates across the country and the world. The fears of Generation Z may be more amorphous than those of the baby boomers, because ostensibly any person could carry out an irrational, violent act at any time.

Coming-of-age experiences are the lens through which people will process subsequent events, including the COVID-19 crisis. Therefore, responses to the pandemic might be strikingly different across generations, as occurs between the baby boomers and Generation Z. Because baby boomers have been alive longer and their brains have absorbed and processed a greater number of experiences, they will likely evaluate risks differently because of their age, prioritizing caution over risk. Generation Z, by contrast, has not lived as long and their brains have not absorbed and processed as many experiences, around 50 years' fewer than baby boomers. Therefore, the Generation Z cohort responds with a willingness to take on more risk, which is developmentally typical.

So, armed with these six principles, what can you do to manage in this time of COVID-19? *Imagine* how lives are affected across ages and generations. *Reflect* on how your coming-of-age experiences have influenced your own response. *Trust* that you can adapt. *Convey* understanding of what people in other stages of the lifespan are going through. *Use* this experience to inform your next crisis experience. *Seek* to gain something, in spite of the losses. We are all capable of change in a crisis, and understanding this can help us confront the ambiguity around the virus, as we navigate it far into the future.

Allyson S. Graf is an assistant professor of psychology who earned her PhD in lifespan psychology from West Virginia University. She trusts in the principles presented in this idea paper because they are grounded in the scientific method and decades of research on lifespan development. Science is not rigid; it recognizes that what we know is ever-changing, fluid, and flexible. When done right, science builds on and embraces new findings that revise how we think about life cycle stages and the impact they have on our lives.

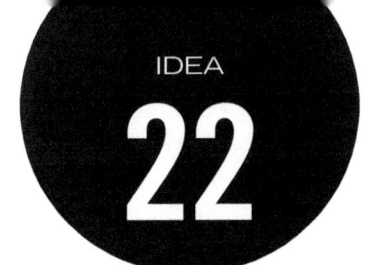

Keep Looking for the Students Who Have Not Connected

Donita Jackson

School Counseling

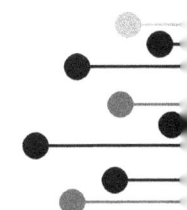

Until the COVID-19 pandemic, elementary and secondary students met almost exclusively face-to-face with school counselors for support with academic challenges, social/emotional concerns, career choices, and college preparation. It was inside office spaces and in hallways that school counselors built relationships with students; learned about their needs, interests, skill sets, and homelife; and encouraged them to make choices that set them up for academic and personal success. It was there that counselors intervened when students were in crisis. Within these school buildings, counselors have acted as conduits of collaboration, bringing together teachers, caregivers, and school administrators to address student needs.

When COVID-19 hit, the country's 285,000 counselors[1] scrambled to replace up close and personal support with virtual meetings. Classroom-based instruction stopped, sending an estimated 55.1 million prekindergarten through 12th-grade students online.[2] Appointments were carried out through videoconferencing, and crises were managed through virtual "calming rooms." Self-care was encouraged through web-guided meditation and mindfulness activities with titles such as "Mindful Moments: 3-Minute Exercises." Tips about how to manage homework and student anxiety were sent to parents in emails. Students who logged in for attendance and to access the day's assignments were asked to rate their stress level, and when they rated it too high, counselors intervened. Counselors helped facilitate "grab and go" events where students and their families picked up free and reduced-priced breakfasts and lunches, care packages, and paper assignments.

While absenteeism was a problem before COVID-19, the pandemic has amplified its magnitude. In one national survey conducted by Educators for Excellence (E4E), teachers of primarily high-income students estimated that 16% were not signing in, attending virtual classes, or doing assignments. Even more concerning, teachers of primarily low-income students reported that 46% were not participating.[3] Schools and school districts also reported that high percentages of students had not responded to text messages or phone calls. A school district in South Carolina reported being unable to contact 800 to 1,100 of the 22,000 students enrolled.[4] A Texas school district reported between 7% and 10% of the district's 67,259 students had been unaccounted for.[5] To make matters worse, the reported rates were likely underestimated.

It was particularly challenging to connect with the almost 20% of students who had no access to computers or the Internet at home. Some schools secured grant money to distribute laptops and equip school buses with Wi-Fi hot spots. Schools also partnered with restaurants and businesses to use their Wi-Fi signals so students could do schoolwork outside or from parked cars. Despite these best efforts, schools lost contact with a significant percentage of students.[6]

As school counselors, we became engulfed in efforts to connect with students and learn why they were not participating in distance learning. Our job was multifaceted and included empathetically encouraging students to establish a routine in the midst of the pandemic while also encouraging teachers to extend deadlines. Our goal was to make sure that all students were engaged at some level while being sensitive to the stresses they were under. Our task was complicated because many of these students knew they could "pass" their courses with minimal effort.

Some students who typically thrived academically and socially struggled to complete even minimal tasks. The uncertainty brought on by the COVID-19 crisis caused paralysis in some students who had previously flourished. The unfortunate reality is that these students lost the motivation and support structure necessary for them to engage.

Many school systems elected to move away from the traditional grading approach of teachers giving assignments, students completing the work, and teachers assigning grades based on performance. Instead, a pass-fail system became commonplace. School administrators chose to adopt this system because they were keenly aware of the many ways the pandemic was disrupting lives. For example, a student we will call Adrian picked up 40-plus work hours a week to supplement his family's income. At the same time, he was also caring for a sick family member at home. Under these strains, he did not log in to access school assignments.

The switch to the pass-fail system, while sensitive to the needs of someone like Adrian, also incentivized other students to put off doing schoolwork: "Why should I put any effort into this?" Some teachers held similar sentiments: "Why put so much effort into planning and preparation when so many students are only doing enough to pass?"

Then there were students, such as one we will call Zoey, who experienced anxiety and depression. Although Zoey had coped with clinical depression for two years before COVID-19, she was skating through her senior year. Many of Zoey's teachers were not even aware of her diagnosis. The isolating impact of the stay-at-home order coupled with the loss of senior year rites of passage sent Zoey in a downward spiral to the point where she was not doing any schoolwork. It was very difficult for her to get out of bed and function, especially early in the pandemic.

In response to these issues, we established a system that enabled teachers to alert counselors to the students who were not engaging. It was through this system that we learned about a student we will call Ava who was not doing her schoolwork. Before COVID-19, Ava was engaged in school, thrived in the classroom, and avidly participated in after-school activities. Why was she not tuned in? When we finally connected with her, we learned that Ava was responsible for guiding a younger elementary-aged sibling. Ava made sure her sibling was present at the biweekly videoconferencing sessions with classmates and helped her access online resources. Because their mother worked longer hours, Ava took on the responsibilities of preparing meals and caring for a grandparent who also lived in the home. When she was able to finally focus on her own work, she felt defeated because she had missed so many assignments.

After conversations with Adrian's, Zoey's, and Ava's teachers, we set up flexible schedules that allowed these students to manage their work more easily. All three students were able to be successful as evidenced by completing the necessary assignments. The stories of Adrian, Zoey, and Ava are concrete examples of how connecting with students changed the course of their quarter.

Still, school counselors often felt overwhelmed and exhausted working to track down students who had seemingly disappeared. And our relationships with students did not end when school concluded for summer break. The widely publicized murders of Ahmaud Arbery, Breonna Taylor, George Floyd, and Rayshard Brooks added another set of concerns and challenges to what students were facing. Protests and unrest brewed across the country as people seeking racial equity and justice converged. With the heightened awareness of and attention to the Black Lives Matter movement, the school opened supportive, safe spaces to convene an affinity group for Black-appearing students so they could share their mental and emotional states.

One student we supported during this crisis is a person we will call Lily, whose mother appears white and father appears Black. By the roll of the genetic dice, her brother appears Black while she appears white. During an affinity group meeting, Lily expressed a need to grieve and protest but felt that her white appearance stood in the way of her full participation. In the session, the group was sensitive to her situation and, in an effort to normalize her feelings, encouraged her to realize that using her voice to speak to white-identifying people is significant. In some situations, people may hear her differently than they would hear those with darker skin.

The stresses of the pandemic are extremely high and working to address them is draining. But in the end, the rewards of connecting with students outweigh the stresses. The thing that keeps school counselors and other educators motivated is our knowledge and belief that when an issue presents itself, such as disengagement, it is the tip of the iceberg. There is almost always a good reason for the behavior. It is our job to try to identify and remedy, if possible, the reason for disengagement just as we did for Adrian, Zoey, and Ava.

To be clear, we know that we are not able to effectively reach every student that disengages during the pandemic. However, we are driven by the idea that there is a reason for the disengagement, and as school counselors, we are compelled to follow the guidelines for serving our students. The call to action is to keep searching for disconnected students and find out why they are not showing up.

If you are a college student reading this, you may be thinking this call applies only to school counselors and not to you. But the challenges of staying connected extend into the college arena, too. Just as counselors look out for their students, college students can take notice of peers who are not connecting and reach out with understanding. Remember that there is always a good reason for their behavior. Think of the things you would say to them face-to-face in class ("How's the paper going?" and "Want to study together for the test?"), and ask these same questions virtually. Your gesture may be the one action that reengages that student. It may take some effort for you, but it is worth the benefits of staying connected when we have to be apart.

Donita Jackson earned her MS degree in school counseling from Xavier University and later completed the Certificate for Advanced Graduate Studies in Professional Counseling at the University of Cincinnati. An energetic and caring listener with over 27 years of experience working with young people as a teacher, coach, and advisor, Jackson currently serves as a high school and college counselor. She trusts that as people are able to integrate new information into their worldview, they can better understand and empathize with one another. For the past few years, her efforts have been intentionally directed toward encouraging student voices in matters of equity and inclusion.

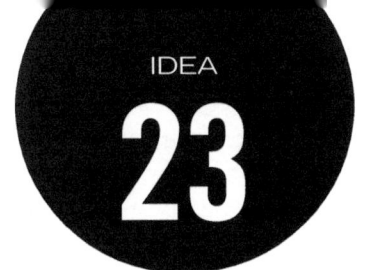

Learn How Trauma Impacts Us

La Shanda Sugg

Trauma Studies

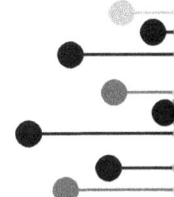

In the broadest sense, trauma can be defined as psychological distress resulting from a disturbing or life-threatening event. Perceptions of danger in our relationships and social experiences trigger survival responses. The coronavirus is a global-scale trauma that has thrown countless people into survival mode as they face threats to their physical health, financial viability, and overall well-being. Likewise, quarantining—whether keeping us apart from loved ones or imprisoning us with an abusive person—can elicit feelings of danger and uncertainty about what lies ahead.

Trauma studies places trauma at the center of self-analysis. The guiding question is not "What's wrong with you?" but rather "What happened to you?" and "What did you do to survive?" People are encouraged to recognize that the problems they have in relationships and life can be traced to the effects of traumatic experiences.

When faced with threat and danger, the brain and body collaborate to automatically generate defense responses to ensure survival and prevent pain. These responses are controlled by the subcortical (or survival) parts of the brain that are outside of conscious control. Defense responses are not decisions that we choose to make or have time to think through; they happen without our permission. That is, our mind and body shift into a state that makes social engagement difficult. For example, imagine driving your car on the highway while talking to a friend when suddenly the driver in front of you slams on the brakes. Acting instinctively, you slam on your brakes. Your heart rate accelerates, you grip the steering wheel tighter. You forget where you are or what time it is. Did you *think* to act in these ways? No. Your brain automatically dispatched the necessary chemicals and signals to let your body know what it had to do to survive.

When stay-at-home orders were announced, can you think of an urge that came over you? It might be running to the store to get toilet paper, food, or disinfectant supplies; withdrawing money from the bank; drinking alcohol; buying a gun; or obsessing over social media posts about the pandemic.

All human survival responses fall into a defense-fear cascade of flock, flight-fight, freeze, and faint. Depending on how the COVID-19 pandemic affects us individually, we have likely engaged in some of these reactions. If we can learn to identify and understand them, we can more skillfully evaluate our responses and care for ourselves and others in the most stressful of times.

Flocking is the first of our defense responses. We are biologically driven to flock, or to seek safety with others. Nature gives us countless examples of organisms finding safety in numbers. Gazelles flock because a lion cannot attack an entire herd; the predator can attack only one gazelle at a time. Flocking among humans can be as simple as a family huddling together during a thunderstorm or college students gathering at the beach in defiance of the COVID-19 pandemic. Humans are hardwired to connect with others; our survival depends on it. Our flock response drives us to be near those we consider safe. Amid social distancing restrictions, we look for ways to flock, such as by virtual meetings on videoconferencing platforms, by phone to check on our loved ones, or even in our imaginations by looking through old photos.

When in a threatening situation, the body mobilizes for a flight or fight response. Interestingly, both types of responses cause our heart to race, pupils to dilate, and muscles to tense as we prepare to either run from or combat the danger. The first instinct is to attempt to flee. Flight is an action taken to gain distance from the situation we perceive as unsafe. We can take flight physically by leaving or running away, by emotionally removing ourselves, or by ignoring that which threatens us. Refusing to answer a telephone call or return a text message is also a form of gaining distance. Flight can also take the form of going out alone for a walk or drive, turning on music, or writing in a journal. During the COVID-19 crisis, the sight of someone in the distance coming toward us can prompt some of us to take flight.

When there is no way to gain distance through flight, we fight. Fight is assertively protecting oneself against a threat, whether real or perceived. Fight responses can include kicking, punching, spitting, verbal aggression, and other acts of defiance; however, the fight response is not always overtly aggressive. People can muster sheer will and determination to fight against a difficult situation or an injustice. They may fight hunger by delivering bags of food, file a lawsuit to keep open or reopen a business, or refuse to wear a face mask. Those who have lost their source of income may grab their guns—sometimes weapons of war—and march to state capitols to protest lockdowns or fight to have businesses reopened.

Freeze is a flight or fight response put on hold. During the freeze response, we experience heightened attentiveness and enhanced vigilance, which prepares us to spring into action when an opportunity presents itself. That sudden stop you make when you are walking down the street and cannot determine if what you see is a long, dirty piece of fabric or a snake is an example of the freeze response. During COVID-19, freeze responses reflect a kind of attentive immobility where, for example, a person may watch the news daily but remain overwhelmed and immobile, or even paralyzed, when it comes to taking action.

When an opportunity to move into action does not come, we move into the faint response. Faint is characterized by absolute immobility, helplessness, or shutdown. We are unable to act. We are susceptible to commands about how to think and behave. This state generates feelings of hopelessness, terror, numbness, dissociation, and collapse. When survival is predicated on submitting or acquiescing to demands, we comply. Over 15 years ago, I was robbed by two men while leaving my restaurant job. I was alone with no one to flock with. I could not outrun or overcome them. So when the robbers demanded my purse, cell phone, and keys, I automatically complied to ensure my survival; I was in a faint response. Only after the robbers left did I regain self-awareness. I began to breathe deeply and recover my senses. My mouth tasted bitter, and my skin felt cold. I became aware again of what I was seeing, smelling, and hearing. Some people exhibited faint responses during COVID-19 that included numbness and shutdown, manifested as sleeping excessively, binge watching TV, or just staring into space.

Our survival responses are situational and depend heavily on previous experiences that have threatened us. A person growing up in a neighborhood where large community parties and fireworks are common may rush to look out a window when they hear a loud bang (flock). A person who grew up in a neighborhood with gun violence may rush away from the window and hit the floor upon hearing these sounds (flight). If we are unaware of patterns in the way we perceive and respond to threats, we will continue to perpetuate them, not realizing we are doing so. The good news is that we can learn to recognize and assess our survival response patterns. While survival responses are automatic, we do have the ability to control them. When we perceive danger or a threat to our safety, we can learn safer ways to respond.

Exploring past events in which we responded with flock, flight or fight, freeze, or faint can help us understand why we lean more heavily toward one or more of the survival responses. Every life experience puts a book in our "mental library." This library houses countless implicit memories, such as riding a bike, taking the same route to work, or remembering the words to a song you have not heard in years. Implicit memories—conscious or unconscious—of a past experience, such as having our car rear-ended, compels us to look into our rearview mirror anytime we make a sudden stop. Our mental library unconsciously weighs every moment as it happens against previous experiences that left us feeling unsafe, as well as against those that brought us security. Because past experiences of feeling safe or unsafe directly determine how we perceive threat and danger, we must be mindful not to judge other people's responses without knowing what books are in their mental libraries.

We can ease the afflictions of this pandemic. Let us remember during the uncertain times of the COVID-19 crisis that we are all humans attempting to stay alive, stay safe, and avoid pain. Our humanity is our common denominator—a foundation from which greater understanding, empathy, and compassion can grow. As we make responses, we can consider what experiences we hold in our mental libraries that drive them. Before making uninformed assumptions about how others are responding, we can extend grace. We can shift from condemnation to curiosity. To help lean toward empathy, ask yourself, "What need is that person's action meeting for them?" If we view people's responses to COVID-19 as attempts to survive and stay safe (physically, emotionally, socially, and financially), we can become less condemning and more kind. In turn, people are more likely to reconsider their actions when others try to understand.

La Shanda Sugg is a licensed professional counselor and certified trauma-responsive therapist who helps families, couples, and individuals understand and heal from their developmental and relational traumas. She is a consultant with the Mourning the Creation of Racial Categories project. Sugg trusts in the importance of learning how trauma impacts us because there is compelling research showing that trauma stays in the body and is associated with lasting changes in the brain. Traumatic stress is associated with increased cortisol and norepinephrine levels when subsequent stressors trigger memories of past traumas. The effects of trauma are understood not only through laboratory research but through observing the lived experiences of humans everywhere. Over the last 10 years she has worked in community mental health with individuals with mental and emotional disorders.

Visualize Social Issues

Robert Del Tredici

Visual Arts

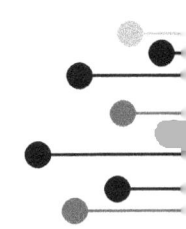

Visual arts is a field of study that encompasses many art forms, including painting, drawing, printmaking, sculpture, ceramics, photography, video art, and filmmaking.[1] As a visual artist, I draw and take photographs.[2] I use the art of photography to address the most pressing social issues. I take photographs with the intent of inspiring people to engage with global issues that are hard for them to wrap their heads around. I use photographs to present issues close-up and to capture the point of view of those most directly affected. My photographs serve as a guide to bring visibility to social issues. I believe in the power of this art form "to help people not only get to know and understand something with their minds but also to feel it emotionally and physically" and to "motivate people to turn thinking into doing."[3]

The pandemic is all around us, but the virus behind the destruction is mostly invisible. Millions worldwide have been sickened by it. Still, an act of the imagination is required to capture it bobbing, weaving, flowing, slowing, hiding, spiking, and making its way. So why should we bring art to bear on this intimate, intricate, wild, worldwide crisis? Because art can shed light on the physical and emotional (and personal) experiences of people, the economic and social turmoil of the disease, and our responses to the virus.

Where might a photographer start when deciding to tackle—to visualize—the social and economic upheaval of the COVID-19 virus, so overwhelming in its reach and impact? To answer this question, I will take you on my journey to investigate another invisible enemy—the bomb and its deadly radiation that has affected communities around the world.

"The Bomb" is my shorthand term for the sprawling, government-funded, scientific–military industrial complex that produced the first atomic bombs, tested in the Alamogordo Desert of New Mexico, before being dropped by the United States on Nagasaki and Hiroshima, Japan, in 1945. The term encompasses the resulting arsenals and stockpiles of nuclear weapons as the United States and the Soviet Union engaged in a nuclear arms race. The nuclear complex that sustains the U.S. arsenal (6,185 nuclear warheads, including those warheads retired and awaiting dismantlement) and stores waste today is still housed in largely the same facilities involved in their creation and stockpiling. The same technology used to create nuclear weapons has since been applied for the commercial purpose of power production. In the United States, there are 95 waste storage sites in 29 states.

The people who live in or near such communities have been exposed to radiation emitted from mass-production of bombs, nuclear weapons testing, radiation accidents, or direct nuclear attacks. We will later apply the process I used to capture their stories to explore the COVID-19 pandemic.

Starting Point

My best advice is to start where "X" marks the spot. Go to the actual place where the real thing came down. I started my photographic journey at a nuclear power generating station in Pennsylvania, the site of the Three Mile Island accident, the most significant accident at a commercial nuclear power plant in U.S. history. It involved a partial reactor meltdown and a continuous and serious radiation leak that was denied and unmeasured at the time. And why go to such a place? I went to feel the place's spirit. I went hoping that the place might speak to me. Or that I might find a way to speak to it.

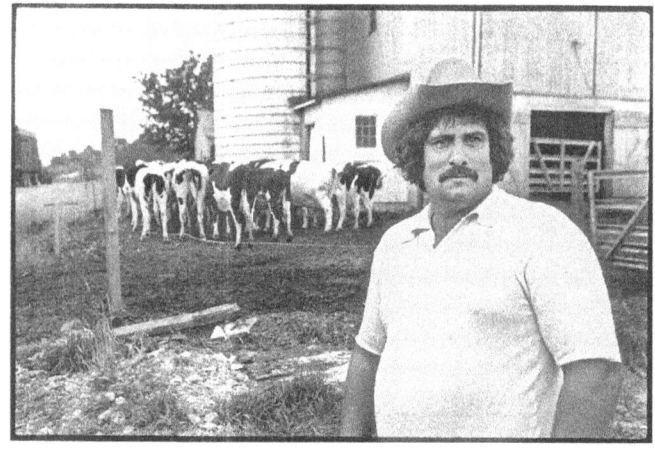

© Robert Del Tredici

Clair Hoover ran a dairy farm in Bainbridge, 5½ miles from the Three Mile Island plant. He demanded answers from the Department of Agriculture after his cattle started aborting and dying one week after the accident. In all, he lost seven cows and 13 calves.[4]

When the Three Mile Island nuclear accident happened in March of 1978, I was living in New York City. At first, I had no idea that under my nose was a huge story about radioactivity, meltdowns, and reactors. I have never forgotten the screaming headline I saw one day at a newsstand: NUKE LEAK OUT OF CONTROL. Overnight, it seemed everyone feared the accident would turn into a meltdown and those panicked by this prospect would try to flee Manhattan, their exodus quickly paralyzed by total gridlock as radioactive clouds from Three Mile Island rolled across this East Coast island city.

The accident was declared over in a week. I searched the papers for human interest stories but found only financial analyses of the industry and accounts of mechanical failures at the plant. I thought maybe I should visit this island of three miles and photograph the survivors. The next morning, I awoke to the vision of a small cloud above my bed, with a finger pointing out of it and a voice that only I could hear, saying, "Go to Three Mile Island." It sounded like a good idea.

I arrived in Middletown, Pennsylvania, on the east side of the Susquehanna River, four miles from the crippled reactor. I had been expecting the scent of annihilation and sickened, rattled townsfolk; but everything looked normal. I asked a man on his front porch what kind of damage he had seen.

He said, "The worst was from all those foreign journalists who trampled on everybody's flowers." He added, "As for me, actually, I put my faith in the Man Upstairs."

That same evening, I met a farmer who would introduce me to dairy farmers, veterinarians, fishermen, nurses, engineers, and retirees over the weeks and months to come. They spoke of holes in leafy trees, rashes on faces, the taste of metal in the mouth, aborting cows and dying calves, bird die-offs, stillborn lambs and still-born human babies, and a color photograph of a two-headed calf.

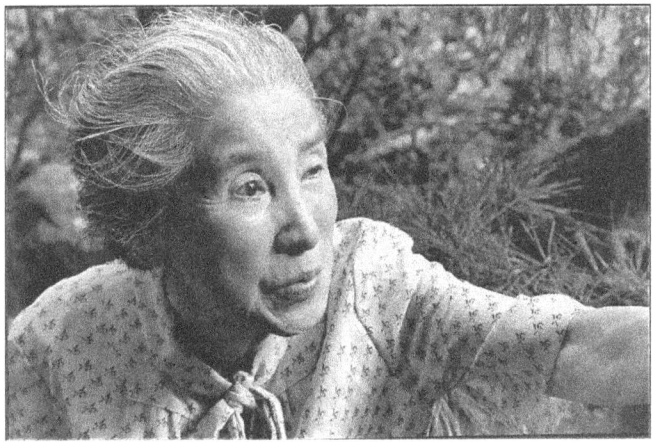

© Robert Del Tredici

I also met mayors, doctors, government officials, a Lutheran preacher, an epidemiologist, an anthropologist, a high-school football coach, and a roomful of fourth graders. I had come to the area to photograph those who had survived the accident. But as I was leaving, I realized that the accident had not happened just to *them*; it had happened to *us*—to the planet.[5]

This experience of documenting the aftermath of the Three Mile Island accident brought keenly into focus my concerns for the environment and my interest in the elusive workings of the human mind. In the process, I found out that the Three Mile Island disaster had behaved unlike any other radiation accident before it,[6] and its effects will be with us for a long time to come. I had entered into the record what the people said and felt and looked like. It set me on the path to record the stories of other radiation-plagued communities.

At Three Mile Island, the shifty, knotted nature of radioactivity had gotten my attention. I felt it was urging me to go deeper. I soon realized what to do next: document the U.S. nuclear weapons complex. If one slightly used commercial reactor could turn people's lives inside out the way the accident on Three Mile Island had done, what must it be like living in the shadow of those top-secret military reactors that had been making plutonium for bombs for over 30 years? I was not as interested in the bomb's might as I was in its "weak force"—the invisible radioactivity emanating from bomb materials, embedded in its residues and shining from its leaks, scattered by its accidents, and living just about forever in its many forms of waste resulting from its mass-production processes.

Still, I was not yet ready to go knocking on bomb-factory doors. Instead, I went to Hiroshima and visited with survivors of the 1945 atomic bombing, listened to their stories, and then I told them my idea. The first time I shared this, an 85-year-old woman, a survivor, told me, "Yes, you *must* do this." At that moment, I became ready to knock on doors.

Tsue Hayashi's 15-year-old daughter died after the U.S. dropped an atomic bomb on the city of Nagasaki, Japan, on August 9, 1945. Her mother described the search for her daughter, Kayoko: "The morning after the bomb, and every day after that, from early morning until evening, I walked all over the city looking for Kayoko. I saw many people suffering and dying. It was very sad. I felt deeply the severe power of the A-bomb. I cannot remember seeing a single other person walking."

The Bomb

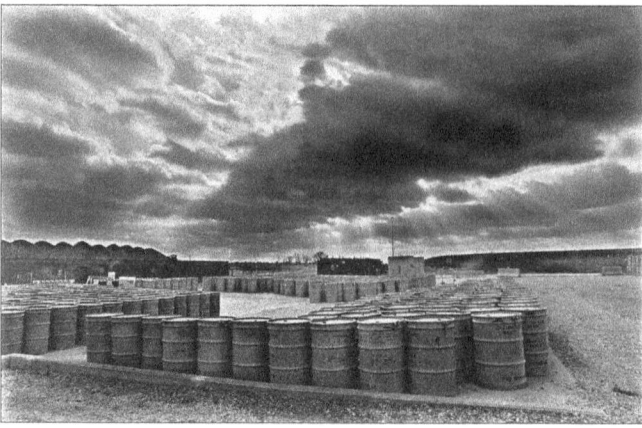

Transuranic Waste Storage Pads, E Area Burial Grounds, Savannah River Site, South Carolina, January 7, 1994. Drums of transuranic waste sit in temporary storage on cement pads designed to diminish the chance the wastes will leak into soil. These wastes are contaminated with plutonium from nuclear weapons mass-production. More than 300,000 such drums are stored or buried throughout the U.S. Plutonium has a half-life of 24,000 years, which means it will remain hazardous for hundreds of thousands of years. When I saw the "Biblical sky" overhead, I could almost hear God saying, "Let there be cleanup."

May 20, 1979

In the 1980s, there were 12 different factories making materials and parts for the hydrogen bomb. I shot aerials over each and talked my way inside seven bomb factories, explaining to public relations officials that I did not want to photograph anything top secret that I should not be shooting, but I did want to take pictures of things that would be alright to shoot. I knew that most of the things inside these factories had not been classified as top secret. I had success with this approach. It was all quite straightforward. What was more difficult for me was to come to terms with the bomb itself.

Nuclear weapons designer Ted Taylor told me two things about the bomb: It was "spherically evil"—that is, no good no matter how you look at it—and that it was highly addictive. I took his words to heart, but I still could not wrap my mind around The Bomb. Then I came up with the idea of visualizing it not as a device but as a sheer cliff face that had me at its base, with no timeline or agenda, inhaling its invisible qualities at a glacial pace. After 3 years, something happened—the cliff face became transparent, and I felt I was on the inside of this enormous entity rather than looking at its unlit façade from without. I felt I had stumbled onto a principle that went something like this: When facing an impossible evil, go deep, stay blank, do not hate, hold tight. This was not exactly a "call to action," but it opened me up enough to take the kinds of action I needed to take. I spent 6 years documenting bomb factories.[7]

Postscript

When the Soviet Union collapsed and closed cities became open, I felt it was time to go photograph things related to the Soviet bomb. I signed up for activist trips, visiting cities[8] around the Mayak plutonium plant whose five reactors and one reprocessing facility had created plutonium for the first Soviet bomb. Lavrentiy Beria, who had directed the construction of the plant and led the Soviet bomb project, ordered the Mayak plant to dump its high-level liquid reprocessing wastes into the nearby Techa River. This dumping went on for 3 years. Lining the banks of the river were 39 villages. This waste-disposal program wiped out 23 of them and created havoc in the minds and bodies of those who remained. None among them knew the reason for their health calamities.

In 1992, I visited the area with a group of activists, and we spent the day in Muslyumovo, the biggest village on the Techa River. After 40 years of silence, this community heard on that day what had been ruining the health of its people. I photographed four Tatar-Bashkir women watching activists measure radioactivity in their river (the surface water came in at 100 times higher than background). With 23 years of nuclear photography behind me, I had photographed the four women in a split second.

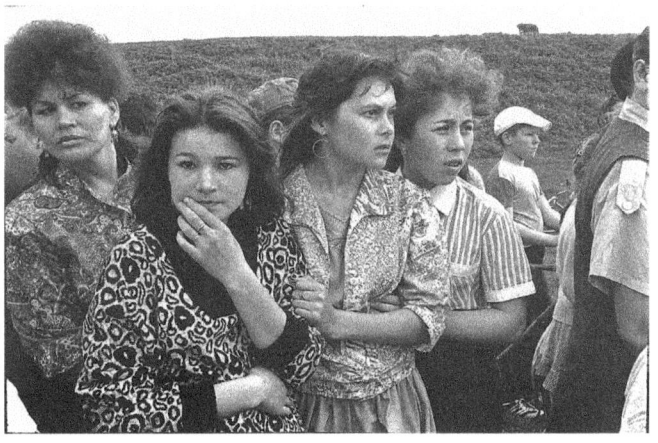

Women from the village of Muslyumovo in the Southern Ural Mountains stand on the banks of the Techa River watching as Westerners measure radiation levels in the water of the river that flows past their town, May 23, 1992.

When I look at the picture, I read in the women's faces grave curiosity, deadly enlightenment, and lethal betrayal. They reminded me of many others, myself included, along with activists, nuclear workers, whistleblowers, atomic veterans, downwinders, meltdown victims, and Hiroshima survivors, who had also been stunned to learn the true price of the nuclear age. I was gratified that this image met my standards for a good picture by breaking through the constraints of its local setting and becoming iconic. That is the transformation I aim for in my art.

Call to Action

If I were to document our pandemic using photographs, I would follow the same guiding principles as when I documented the bomb. First, I would go to "X" marks the spot, where the real thing came down.[9] I would go to feel the spirit of the places, hoping that the places might speak to me. And I would try to find a way to speak to them.

In this pandemic we have more than 185,000 dead Americans and counting. I have not seen any sign of them dying; they died alone without friends and family. How can this be? Seeing the dying is important. How might we see? I would look for ways to visit hospitals, churches, morgues, cremation sites, and graveyards. I would try to find ways to attend ritual scatterings of ashes. I would likely be denied access at some or all of these places. But that is the thing about going to the "X": You never know what will happen.

One thing I know for sure: I would photograph faces. There are always faces. I would capture faces of nurses, doctors, health workers, preachers.

And because Black Lives Matter street demonstrations have been braided into the pandemic, I would go for portraits of nonviolent sitters and marchers, and also looters. I would take close-ups of those police officers in Washington, DC, at demonstrations wearing generic riot gear with no lettering identifying who they were. I would also go after the officers in riot gear standing still and silently staring through helmeted face shields. I would go up to each one and make a portrait featuring their eyes on the other side of that great plastic divide.

In the end, I would be happy if, out of all the photographs I took, I came away with three good shots. These are the externals. To approach the internal realm, I would sit long in silence with the peaceful protesters. If families would allow, I would sit with them as their loved ones lay dying apart from them. I would look for what poets and essayists have been saying. And I would not mention the president of the United States. And I would avoid clichés like the plague.

For starters, these are some of the things I would do. How about you? What would you do?

Robert Del Tredici is a photographer and artist who has been teaching photography, cinema history, and the art of animated film since the 1970s. He trusts in his process of learning from the people who experience crises directly, including the people in the trenches. This is the best way art represents an experience. He has been documenting the nuclear age since 1979. He co-founded The Atomic Photographers Guild in 1987. Del Tredici has exhibited his portraits and documentary work in London, Hiroshima, Washington, DC, Hong Kong, and other cities. In the 1970s and 1980s, he studied under Tibetan teacher Chogyam Trungpa, who gave him the name "Good Eye of Enlightenment." The Special Collections and University Archives of the W. Frank Steely Library at the Northern Kentucky University has the world's largest collection of Del Tredici's Moby Dick–related art.

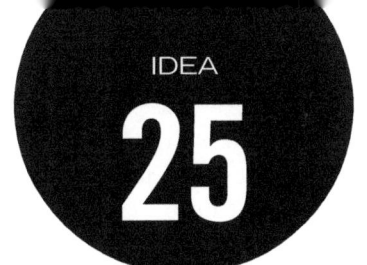

Learn How Another Culture Responds to Crises

Bo-Kyung Kim Kirby

World Languages

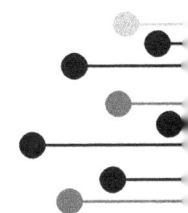

Departments of world languages offer courses and opportunities to learn about languages, literatures, and cultures, with the goal of increasing language proficiency and communication. One benefit of knowing more than one language is that it opens the door to conversations with more people around the world. But knowledge of other languages can also help you think in different ways, see things from new perspectives, and in some cases, lead you to make different decisions.

Many people across the globe are fortunate to grow up in a multilingual environment, and they become native speakers of more than one language. Others may acquire another language later in life, which requires conscious effort and study. The effort and study of learning a language offers opportunities to think carefully about the language and its cultural context. Even small points of grammar can have broad implications.

Here is one example from the Korean language, which I teach to college students. Suppose you want to say "My mother is hungry." In Korean you say *"Uri eomeoni sijanghaseyo."*

The word "eomeoni" (mother) is straightforward. But the other two words carry a lot of significance that may surprise English speakers. The word "uri" does not actually mean "my"; it means "our." The Korean language has other words specifically for "my." So a literal reading of that sentence is *"Our* mother is hungry." But suppose you insist: I am an only child! I want to say *"my* mother," not *"our* mother" in Korean. In theory, you could say very literally "My mother is hungry," but a Korean hearing this would feel that was very wrong. Similarly, a Korean would never say "my country"; they would say "our country." This gives us some insight into how Koreans focus on group identity.

The word "sijanghaseyo" (is hungry) can only be used when it is an "honored" person who is hungry. This could be your mother or another elder or the president of your company, for example. A different word for "is hungry" is used for yourself or your friends: *paegophayo.* But this word would sound very wrong if you used it for your mother. This tells us a bit more about how Koreans think of respect.

This one sentence, then, illustrates two points. First, Korea is a culture of respect. Second, it has a very strong focus on the group over the individual. But what does this imply in times of crisis, such as in the COVID-19 pandemic?

Many people ask me about South Korea's handling of COVID-19. A number of stories have been written about this success, with titles such as "What's Behind South Korea's COVID-19 Exceptionalism?"[1] The first cases of COVID-19 were reported in the United States and South Korea on the same day (January 20, 2020). Within a few months, South Korea had been widely praised as a model for handling the virus, including by the World Health Organization. The numbers of infected people and the death rates were lower, and the numbers of people tested were notably higher than in other countries. Korea quickly provided high-tech mass testing, free to anyone who came into contact with someone who showed symptoms. And for those who tested positive, their contacts were digitally and securely traced and tested. The country even pioneered the soon widespread drive-through testing and "phonebooth testing,"[2] and took concerted steps to balance privacy and public health concerns around such testing.[3] It also quickly implemented preventative measures such as school closures, social distancing, and face mask campaigns.

At the same time, South Korea, its provinces, and its cities were *not* locked down. People who had no evidence of contact with a case of COVID-19 and who had no symptoms were never ordered to quarantine. However, arrivals from out of the country were ordered to do so. Businesses and buildings remained open if a COVID-19-positive person had not been inside. People also did not have a problem with empty shelves of daily-use products at stores. The country even managed to successfully hold a parliamentary election.

How was this possible when most countries did not attain this degree of success in the early months of the pandemic? One factor was Korea's prior experience with pandemics. In 2015, Korea was hit strongly by the MERS (Middle East respiratory syndrome) virus. Within two months after the first patient was identified, more than 16,000 people were quarantined, 186 were infected, and 38 died. At the beginning of this period, the government could not control the virus and also withheld details so as to not cause public anxiety. A large, prominent hospital deliberately hid the case of one of their doctors, who later became a superspreader. Each error was followed by another error. In the end, the government had to apologize for their egregious mismanagement. They promised, "Next time we will be prepared."

Another factor that contributed to their exceptional management of the pandemic was Korea's unprecedented push for government transparency in the wake of the impeachment of their president in 2017 for abuse of power. That president is now serving a 20-year prison sentence.[4] The national outcry against corruption was so huge that the incoming presidential administration had to rebuild public trust from scratch. And this new focus on accountability, in a country that was highly autocratic one generation ago (and a dictatorship two generations ago), put the country in a better place to respond to a crisis. While lessons learned about public health preparedness and political change were crucial to Korea's pandemic response, success ultimately relies on human behavior. And that is where language and culture come in.

In the language example above, we saw that Koreans value certain notions of respect and group identification. As a person, you are valued more as part of a group than alone as an individual. If you go to a restaurant or bar after work with your coworkers, you are careful to act just like the others. You do not want to stand out, and you do not want to not join in. Your life is filled with multiple group bonds: your coworkers, your fellow school alumni (even elementary school alumni), and of course, your family. These groups are all knitted together. It is a culture not of "me" but of "us." Some features of group-focused culture that protect against virus transmission are described below.

Do you dare not wear a face mask? Of course not, because everybody is wearing one. Even before the onset of COVID-19, wearing masks outside the home was common practice in large cities such as Seoul, where air quality can be low and where fine, yellow dust particles are carried in the wind from the Gobi Desert. With face masks a familiar sight for all Koreans, increased adoption during the pandemic was easy to achieve.

What about social distancing? Although hugs and handshakes have become popular, the traditional greeting is a bow.

What about a program on your mobile phone that tracks your location to control the spread of disease? Is that an invasion of your privacy? If you are a Korean you might ask, "What privacy?" In groups, everyone knows everyone else's business. Privacy is common in cultures that value individualism; this characteristic is less prominent in Korean culture.

But one interesting exceptional case in which privacy was protected arose during the pandemic. The matter related to those Koreans going to gay clubs and bars. LGBTQ culture is still stigmatized in some parts of Korean culture, and people going to these clubs must often take care to hide it from their employers or families. So the government adopted contact tracing practices that anonymize and secure data so that those in the LGBTQ community could be free to report any health-relevant contacts without worry of this information being disclosed.

Another interesting thing about South Korea's response to the pandemic is that food fads and myths tend to propagate quickly and uncritically.[5] For example, it is widely believed that kimchi, the fermented cabbage side dish that is Korea's best known food, can fight coronaviruses or at least strengthen immunity against them.

In the end, the way countries respond to crises is a function of culture as much as history and politics. When we learn another language as an adult, we do not unquestioningly absorb all the cultural assumptions and practices behind the words as we would if learning as a child. Childhood is the time when we learn both the language and culture simultaneously. But as adults, we can still learn much about a culture through our own effort, and we can see how language mirrors and supports group versus individual responses to crises. When you know another language, you can critique your own and your culture's response. You can see there is another way.

Bo-Kyung Kim Kirby is a writer, translator, and instructor of Korean language and computer programming. She earned her master's degree in Korean literature from Kyunghee University in Seoul and did additional graduate studies in computer science from Wayne State University. She trusts the idea that language is a window into culture and responses people make. She bases this trust on the experience of living in both Korea and the United States and being fluent in both languages. Kim Kirby knows that words are more than words, because they bring with them a host of associations. As a translator, she is in a unique position that requires her to quickly understand the layers of cultural associations and meanings that words carry. Translators serve as a bridge between two cultures and they must make snap decisions about how much cultural information to include in the translation.

Notes

Preface

[1] In a Pew survey, 12% of adults said their personal lives have "stayed about the same" since this coronavirus outbreak, whereas 44% said their lives have changed "in a major way." See Pew Research Center. (2020, March 30). Most Americans say the coronavirus outbreak has impacted their lives. https://www.pewsocialtrends.org/2020/03/30/most-americans-say-coronavirus-outbreak-has-impacted-their-lives/

[2] U.S. Census Bureau. (2020). *Educational attainment. American Community Survey 2018: ACS 1-year estimates subject tables* (Table ID: S1501). https://data.census.gov/cedsci/table?q=S1501&tid=ACSST1Y2018.S1501

[3] Simultaneous with lockdowns, colleges and universities across the country launched fundraising campaigns to support students in need.

[4] Each idea paper does not speak for the entire discipline; each is one voice among many. A great exercise in any course would be to ask students to write such a paper in response to the pandemic using one idea from the class.

[5] If your discipline is not represented here, we did not intentionally leave it out. It came down to who was able to do this during a time of great upheaval when face-to-face classes transitioned to online platforms with no notice.

[6] Of course, there are many generous reviewers. But it is the most mean-spirited reviewers that have us agonizing over every piece we write.

[7] When we say a surprising amount of time, that includes the time each author spent settling on the idea to present and writing the draft; the time the 11 reviewers spent reading each paper, flagging the best and most elusive paragraphs; and the time four editors dedicated to synthesizing the reviews and then offering concrete suggestions and edits. Each idea paper went back to the author for two additional rounds after the initial draft. And, finally, the time the copy editor took to check for inconsistencies and improve readability both midway through and at the end of the process.

[8] Fitzgerald, F. S. (1925). *The great Gatsby*. Charles Scribner's Sons.

The Need for Reader Advocates

[1] Postman, N. (1986). *Amusing ourselves to death; Public discourse in the age of show business*. Heinemann.

1. Know That Things Are Not What They Seem (Sociology)

[1] There are levels of social forces. In this paper, we named what we might call *immediate social forces*, but these are shaped by other social forces. Whether you have a grocery store in the heart of your neighborhood is shaped by a capitalist system intent to put stores near high-income households. If the racial composition of your neighborhood is of only one race, we can say that this neighborhood has not recovered from another social force—400 years of enforced segregation. There are many social forces behind how COVID-19 affects your neighborhood, but many of those forces have to do with the extent to which your neighborhood is interconnected with the world (i.e., Is it rural or urban? Is there an international airport nearby? Is it near a university?).

[2] Sociologist Peter Berger (2011) coined the phrase "Things are not what they seem." He wrote, "The fascination of sociology lies in the fact that its perspective makes us see in a new light the very world in which we have lived all our lives. . . . It can be said that the first wisdom of sociology is things are not what they seem" (pp. 21, 23). Berger, P. L. (2011). *Invitation to sociology: A humanistic perspective*. Open Road Media.

[3] Individuals' resources vary widely depending on age, race, gender, social class, and other key identifiers.

[4] Sociologist Robert K. Merton (1996) wrote about anticipated and unanticipated consequences. He called anticipated consequences *manifest* and unanticipated consequences *latent*. For the purposes of this paper, we use the terms *anticipated and unanticipated responses*. After all, people's responses do have consequences. For more, see Merton, R. K. (1996). *On social structure and science*. University of Chicago Press.

[5] One example of people finding a "best" option in a traumatic situation comes from the research of sociologists Amith Ben-David and Yoav Lavee (1992). Their research on ways Israeli families responded in a time of crisis is instructive. Specifically, the researchers studied how families responded to missile attacks on their homes launched by Iraqi military. The families took cover in sealed rooms and put on gas masks. Some families responded in this way: "We laughed, and we took pictures of each other with the gas masks on" or "We

talked about different things, about the war, we told jokes, we heard the announcements on the radio." Other families responded by staying very quiet yet feeling a strong sense of togetherness: "I was quiet, immersed in my thoughts. We were all around the radio. . . . Nobody talked much." Still other families responded in ways that brought tension: "We fought with the kids about putting on their masks, and also between us about whether the kids should put on their masks. There was much shouting and noise." This research illustrates that even under extremely stressful circumstances people can respond in ways that can make things better rather than worse. Ben-David, A., & Yoav, L. (1992). Families in the sealed room: Interaction patterns of Israeli families during SCUD missile attacks. *Family Process, 31*(1), 35–44.

2. Connect and Reconnect With Food (Anthropology)

[1] In the United States, the discipline of anthropology is traditionally divided into what we refer to as the *four subfields*. These focal areas include archaeology (the study of the human past), biological anthropology (the study of humans as biological organisms), linguistics (the study of human languages), and cultural anthropology (the study of contemporary human societies and cultures). Culture is a key concept and unifying theme among the subdisciplines.

[2] I do not discuss disordered eating in any detail in this idea paper. However, there is information emerging about disordered eating in relation to stress and the effects of the COVID-19 lockdown. One source is https://www.bbc.com/worklife/article/20200331-how-to-eat-a-healthy-diet-when-work-from-home-coronavirus.

[3] For examples see the following stories: (1) Davies, E. (2020, March 31). People rush to raise backyard chickens amid egg shortages, coronavirus concerns. *The Washington Post*. https://www.washingtonpost.com/local/people-rush-to-raise-backyard-chickens-amid-egg-shortages-coronavirus-concerns/2020/03/30/b9d4d3ea-71d7-11ea-a9bd-9f8b593300d0_story.html. (2) Robinson, A. (2020, April 5). Vegetable seeds are the new toilet paper. *Modern Farmer*. https://modernfarmer.com/2020/04/vegetable-seeds-are-the-new-toilet-paper/

[4] Stress—such as stress induced by the COVID-19 crisis—can break down the way we consume food. In this case, I am thinking of disordered eating. See Gordon, A. (2020, June 14). *Coronavirus: Living with eating disorders in lockdown*. BBC. https://www.bbc.com/news/uk-northern-ireland-52926525

[5] Bureau of Labor Statistics. (2020, March). *News release: The employment situation*. U.S. Department of Labor. https://www.bls.gov/news.release/archives/empsit_04032020.pdf

[6] Zilber, A. (2020, April 6). Stark photos show miles-long rows of cars waiting outside a Florida food bank as demand surges by 600 per cent and more than half-a-million residents file for unemployment. *Daily Mail*. https://www.dailymail.co.uk/news/article-8193153/Miles-long-row-cars-waits-outside-Florida-food-bank-demand-produce-surges-600-cent.html

[7] Newton, C. (2020, April 8). Navajo Nation: Fears of hunger as COVID-19 lockdown to intensify. *Aljazeera News/United States*. https://www.aljazeera.com/news/2020/04/navajo-nation-fears-hunger-covid-19-lockdown-intensify-200407162033892.html

[8] Food experts have argued for decades that poor diet and subsequent diet-related illnesses have made a significant impact on loss of life, well-being, and health care costs. See the *Union of Concerned Scientists'* statement on "Healthy Food for All" at https://www.ucsusa.org/food/healthy-food. See also Macintosh, E. (2017, October 10). *What we eat is making us sick say food experts*. European Environmental Bureau's META. https://meta.eeb.org/2017/10/10/what-we-eat-is-making-us-sick-say-food-experts/

3. Look to Science for Answers (Biology)

[1] To date, seven coronaviruses that infect humans are known: HCoV-229E, HCoV-NL63, HCoV-OC43, HCoV-HKU1, severe acute respiratory syndrome coronavirus (SARS-CoV), Middle East respiratory syndrome coronavirus (MERS-CoV), and SARS-CoV-2 (the cause of COVID-19). For more, see these two sources: https://www.ncbi.nlm.nih.gov/pmc/articles/PMC7098031/ and https://www.cdc.gov/coronavirus/types.html

[2] RNA stands for ribonucleic acid and is a collection of genetic material packed inside a protein shell. RNA is a single-stranded molecule. (In comparison, the DNA molecule is double-stranded.) DNA is stable under alkaline conditions, while RNA is not. The genome size of coronaviruses makes them one of the largest RNA viruses.

[3] I studied biology in the United States, and I now work in a university clinical center in Bosnia. The official name of my country is Bosnia and Herzegovina.

[4] The Nipah (NEE-pa) virus (NiV) is carried by fruit bats living in rural South Asia. Its most serious symptoms are flu and brain inflammation. Infected bats do not get sick, but their saliva and urine can infect pigs, which can then transmit the virus to farmers. The World Health Organization classifies Nipah as a priority

disease, which means there is an urgent need to accelerate research on the virus.

[5] Jabr, F. (2020, April 6). How realistic is *Contagion?* The movie doesn't skimp on science. *New Scientist.* https://www.newscientist.com/article/2239913-how-realistic-is-contagion-the-movie-doesnt-skimp-on-science/

[6] *Contagion* deals with a host of social issues that arise in times of pandemic—conspiracy theorists, a breakdown in social order, missteps by government, quarantines, ethical questions (e.g., Who tests the vaccine?), and scientific debate over the average number of new cases of infections.

[7] Scientists do not believe the new coronavirus came from a lab. The origin of the COVID-19 virus is natural, not man-made. Immunologist Nigel McMillan said, "If you were going to design it in a lab, the sequence changes make no sense, as all previous evidence would tell you it would make the virus worse. No system exists in the lab to make some of the changes found." For more, see Bowler, J. (2020, April 20). Scientists are tired of explaining why the COVID-19 virus was not made in a lab. *Science Alert.* https://www.sciencealert.com/here-s-what-scientists-think-of-the-coronavirus-was-made-in-a-lab-rumour

[8] Just as people can get a cold more than once, they might also show symptoms of COVID-19 more than once.

[9] For surface disinfection, use a 1:50 dilution of bleach in water, but only externally! Please do not inject or ingest bleach into your body because you will get extremely ill and likely die. In that case, COVID-19 is the least of your concerns!

[10] Bromage, E. (2020, May 6). The risks—know them—avoid them. https://www.erinbromage.com/post/the-risks-know-them-avoid-them

[11] To establish this estimate, aerosol scientists employ technology such as laser beams and high-sensitivity cameras that can trap droplet particles in the air as people sneeze, talk loudly, and breathe. For more, see Kay, J. (2020, April 23). COVID-19 superspreader events in 28 countries: Critical patterns and lessons. *Quillette.* https://quillette.com/2020/04/23/covid-19-superspreader-events-in-28-countries-critical-patterns-and-lessons/

4. Work to Become Resilient (Clinical Counseling)

[1] Dorian, E. (1982). *The quality of witness: A Romanian diary 1937–1944* (1st ed.). University of North Carolina Press.

[2] Frankl, V. (1984). *Man's search for meaning: An introduction to logotherapy.* Simon & Schuster.

5. Engage in New Ways (Community Engagement)

[1] The Carnegie Classification of Institutions of Higher Education provides a widely accepted definition of community engagement, available at https://www.brown.edu/swearer/carnegie/about.

[2] Butin, D. (2010). *Service-learning in theory and practice: The future of community engagement in higher education.* Palgrave Macmillan.

[3] The computer science students built a tracking database for Creative Aging, a Cincinnati-based nonprofit that brings artists, performers, and educators to senior centers, retirement communities, adult day care centers, and nursing homes. A full report on the computer science class, CSC 301: Web Programming, is available online at https://inside.nku.edu/civicengagement/programs/mayerson/spring2020/CSC301.html.

6. Slow Down, Pause, Reflect (Creative Writing)

[1] Poetry saved my life. I say that without drama. I had a difficult childhood and hard teenage years. I became pregnant early and kept the child. I almost gave up on education. But then I took a class called American Poetry where Lucille Clifton, Elizabeth Bishop, and Sylvia Plath became a part of my "mouthful of air" (from Yeats's poem "He Thinks of Those Who Have Spoken Evil of His Beloved" in the book *The Wind Among the Reeds,* 1899). I took poetry workshops. I earned a BA, an MA, and an MFA, all in poetry writing. I could make a list of all that poetry has done for me, what I hope it will do for you. But right now, in this moment, we most need to care for ourselves, putting on our own masks before we help those who need to put on theirs. And we can do this by allowing our minds to stop. To pause. Even once per day. So that we can understand how the COVID-19 crisis affects our minds.

[2] Hirsch, E. (1999). *How to read a poem: And fall in love with poetry.* Houghton Mifflin Harcourt.

[3] Reuters. (2020, April 5). *Queen Elizabeth addresses the United Kingdom on coronavirus outbreak.* https://www.reuters.com/article/us-health-coronavirus-britain-queen-text/queen-elizabeths-addresses-the-united-kingdom-on-coronavirus-outbreak-idUSKBN21N0TU

[4] Quote by Simone Weil taken from Waldron, R. (2008). *Thomas Merton: Master of attention: An exploration of prayer* (p. 90). Paulist Press.

[5] Quote by Nicolas Malebranche taken from Hirsch, E. (2000). *How to read a poem and fall in love with poetry.* Houghton Mifflin Harcourt.

[6] Wei, W. (1922, February). A green stream. In H. Monroe (Ed.), *Poetry* (p. 8). https://www.poetryfoundation.org/poetrymagazine/browse?contentId=15508

7. Grasp the Deeper Meaning of Social Distancing (Critical White Studies)

[1] We made the decision to capitalize White and Black in reference to racial categories, identities, and appearances. The *New York Times* recently decided to capitalize Black but not white. We believe that to do this sends the message that White is not a racial category. We do not capitalize white when used in reference to white supremacy or white privilege.

[2] We use the term *classified* because the ideas of race and distinct racial categories are European created. These categories are socially created; they are not the biological/genetic certainty that we are brought up to believe. Also, *classified* reminds us that divisions are arbitrary, not fixed.

[3] This phrase can be found in the poem "That Time I Talked to Race" by Kirsten Hurst in the documentary *The categories Black and White* [Film]. Ferrante, J., & Gray, J. (Directors). (2017). The Mourning the Creation of Racial Categories Project. https://www.ket.org/program/mourning-the-creation-of-racial-categories/

[4] In the United States, Hispanic is officially recognized as an ethnic category, although many people think of it as a racial category.

[5] While the categories named in the idea paper may not correspond to your ideas of what the "races" are, these are the categories the United States officially recognizes today.

[6] Nagle, R. (2020, April 24). Native Americans left out of U.S. coronavirus data and labelled as "other." *The Guardian*. https://www.theguardian.com/us-news/2020/apr/24/us-native-americans-left-out-coronavirus-data

[7] Srikanth, A. (2020, May 11). Doctors Without Borders arrives in New Mexico to help Native Americans battle the coronavirus. *The Hill*. https://thehill.com/changing-america/respect/diversity-inclusion/497132-doctors-without-borders-arrives-in-new-mexico-to

[8] Nagle, R. (2020, April 24). Native Americans left out of U.S. coronavirus data and labelled as "other." *The Guardian*. https://www.theguardian.com/us-news/2020/apr/24/us-native-americans-left-out-coronavirus-data

[9] Lakhani, N. (2020, May 8). Navajo Nation reels under weight of the coronavirus—and history of broken promises. *The Guardian*. https://www.theguardian.com/world/2020/may/08/navajo-nation-coronavirus

[10] Srikanth, A. (2020, May 11). Doctors Without Borders arrives in New Mexico to help Native Americans battle the coronavirus. *The Hill*. https://thehill.com/changing-america/respect/diversity-inclusion/497132-doctors-without-borders-arrives-in-new-mexico-to

[11] The peoples that make up these 2,000 distinct Indian-classified societies responded in different ways to removal policies. All were drawn into a divide-and-conquer strategy that pitted tribes against one another. Some fought to stop intrusion; others appealed to the courts or went to war with each other. Why? Because survival depended on finding a place in an economic system that was destroying them.

[12] The Creek Civil War involved opposing Creek factions, with Spain, Britain, the United States, and the Cherokee supporting the different factions. Jackson, who later became president of the United States, built his reputation on Indian removal.

[13] Centers for Disease Control and Prevention. (2020, June 4). *COVID-19 in racial and ethnic minority groups*. https://www.cdc.gov/coronavirus/2019-ncov/need-extra-precautions/racial-ethnic-minorities.html

[14] To enforce the Jim Crow system, the law needed to determine who was Black and who was White. The legal question: Into which category would a person with one Black-classified parent, grandparent, or great-grandparent fall? The answer varied depending on the state. States classified someone as Black if they had 1/4, 1/8, 1/16, 1/32, or 1/64 "Black" blood, or any perceptible physical evidence of descent from Africa. This shows that people were classified, not inherently Black or White.

[15] X, M., & Haley, A. (2015). *The autobiography of Malcolm X*. Ballantine Books.

8. Change the Story, Change What Is Possible (Cultural Studies)

[1] For an accessible overview of the diverse field of cultural studies, see Barker, C., & Jane, E. A. (2016). *Cultural studies: Theory and practice* (5th ed.). SAGE.

[2] While the story many anthems tell is built out of a series of declamations and imperatives ("God Save Our Queen!"), others, such as the "Star Spangled Banner," are more narrative in structure and even a bit enigmatic. Artist Laurie Anderson describes the U.S. national anthem as "just a lot of questions written during a fire" in Anderson, L. (1990). *Public service announcement: National anthem* [Video]. YouTube. https://www.youtube.com/watch?v=9cE6Pg2q3lI

[3] The term *rags to riches* comes from an influential series of novels written by Horatio Alger in the late 19th century.

[4] The concepts of *dominant*, *residual*, and *emergent* stories were developed in the early 1960s by the British cultural theorist Raymond Williams.

[5] McCort, K. (2020, February 28). Misfits Theater Company flipping the bard on his head with all female, non-binary "Macbeth." *Boulder Daily Camera*. https://www.dailycamera.com/2020/02/28/misfits-theater-company-flipping-the-bard-on-his-head-with-all-female-non-binary-macbeth/

[6] As examples of how dominant stories contain contradictory values and ideas, think of powerful cultural narratives such as the Star Wars or Avengers film series. What values are they reinforcing? Is it a dominant narrative that, when in a crisis, we should look to strong, heroic (and usually white and male) leaders to save us? Or is it that we all need to band together across lines of difference to oppose the forces of tyranny and oppression?

9. Embrace the Math You Thought You Would Never Need
(Developmental Mathematics)

[1] Stokes E. K., Zambrano L. D., Anderson, K. N., Marder, E. P., Raz, K. M., Suad, E. B. F., Tie, Y., & Fullerton, K. E. (2020, June 15). Coronavirus disease 2019 case surveillance—United States, January 22–May 30, 2020 (*Morbidity and Mortality Weekly Report*). Centers for Disease Control and Prevention. http://dx.doi.org/10.15585/mmwr.mm6924e2. Cases updated 9/2/2020.

[2] In an ordered list with an odd number of items (say, 5 people ages 20, 35, 65, 75, and 99), the median age is the number in the middle of the list. In this case, it is 65. If there is an even number of items (4 people ages 20, 65, 75, and 99), the median is the average of the two middle numbers. The average of 65 and 75 makes the median age 70.

[3] Magan, C. (2020, May 31). Most of Minnesota's COVID-19 fatalities also fought other chronic illnesses: Here are the details. *Twin Cities Pioneer Press*. https://www.twincities.com/2020/05/31/most-of-minnesotas-coronavirus-covid-19-fatalities-also-fought-other-chronic-illnesses/

10. Read, Write, Make Meaning
(English Literature)

[1] Douglass published his second autobiography 10 years later, when he was 37 years old. He published his third autobiography in 1892, when he was 74.

11. Don't Blame the Bats
(Environmental Sociology)

[1] Indeed, reports are beginning to confirm those most at risk of dying as a result of COVID-19 are those most vulnerable to environmental stressors of all sorts. In virus hotspots such as New York and Louisiana, death rates were highest among Latino and Black populations. These groups are more likely to live deep in city centers where pollution is most concentrated and so experience underlying lung issues and other associated risk factors for COVID-19 at higher rates than others. This, combined with structural inequalities such as limited access to health care and racism within the health care system (which often leads to symptoms being taken less seriously), has caused disproportionate death rates in communities of color. Poor white communities may also have increased risks related to environmental health exposures. Many have raised concerns about the predominantly white Appalachian region, for example, where there are high rates of black lung among miners, high numbers of people living below the poverty line, and limited access to health care.

[2] Agricultural (as well as industrial) runoff creates "dead zones," areas in oceans and large lakes where marine life has been killed off from reduced levels of oxygen.

[3] Kolbert, E. (2014). *The sixth extinction: An unnatural history*. Picador.

[4] Hannah, R. (2019, November 11). Half of the world's habitable land is used for agriculture. *Our World and Data*. https://ourworldindata.org/global-land-for-agriculture

[5] Sharp, P. M., & Hahn, B. H. (2010). The evolution of HIV-1 and the origin of AIDS. *Philosophical Transactions: Biological Sciences, 365*(1552), 2487–2494. https://www.ncbi.nlm.nih.gov/pmc/articles/PMC2935100/

[6] Quammen, D. (2012). *Spillover: Animal infections and the next human pandemic*. W. W. Norton.

[7] Quammen, D. (2012). *Spillover: Animal infections and the next human pandemic*. W. W. Norton.

[8] World Health Organization. (2020, February 10). *Ebola virus disease*. https://www.who.int/news-room/fact-sheets/detail/ebola-virus-disease

[9] Zoonotic transmission of coronaviruses likely occurred in isolated cases long before the SARS outbreak of 2003 and the COVID-19 outbreak of 2019.

[10] Quammen, D. (2012). *Spillover: Animal infections and the next human pandemic*. W. W. Norton.

[11] Centers for Disease Control and Prevention. (2017, December 6). *Severe acute respiratory syndrome (SARS)*. https://www.cdc.gov/sars/index.html

[12] Chen, F., Cao, S., Xin, J., & Xiaohua, L. (2013). Ten years after SARS: Where was the virus from? *Journal of Thoracic Disease, 5*(2), 152–167.

[13] Humans have not caused equal damage to the environment. Americans, for example, are 5% of the world's population but consume over a third of its resources and produce most of its trash. In a Western cultural tradition that views "human" and "environment" as separate entities, the idea makes sense that if we could remove ourselves from the environment, then Earth might heal itself.

12. See the Predictability in the Chaos of Pandemics (Film Studies)

[1] Epidemics affect a large number of people living in a specific community, population, or region. A pandemic is also an epidemic, but it affects people living in multiple countries or continents.

[2] This phrase comes from Elia Kazan's film *Panic in the Streets* (1950). "Panic in the Streets" was also the title of the first season of films at the National Film Theatre in London that used the term *epidemic cinema* in 1988. That season was curated and documented by Judith Williamson and Mark Finch, who were examining how the AIDS pandemic had been predicted and analyzed in select films.

[3] Indicators are derived from the Williamson-Finch anatomy of epidemic cinema and from my own research and publications. Words and phrases in quotations are from Williamson, J. (1992). *Deadline at dawn: Film writings, 1980–1990*. Marion Boyars.

[4] There is also a database (a work in progress) on my website *Globalization and Film* at https://tzaniello.wordpress.com/ that lists the titles of 104 films of epidemic cinema, with the disease vector or pathogen noted for each film. The database can be used for consultation, viewing, and further analysis. The films listed supplement the examples in this idea paper. Also included are films—none of which are discussed here—from the popular subgenre of epidemic cinema featuring zombies.

[5] See other titles in Wald, P. (2008). *Contagious: Cultures, carriers, and the outbreak narrative*. Duke University Press.

[6] *Mise-en-scène* is a cinematic term meaning "to place on the stage." It includes all the visuals—props, lighting, characters, speech, music, and action—used to make any given shot or sequence in a film.

[7] Semmker, I. A. (1998). Ebola goes pop: The filovirus from literature to film. *Literature and Medicine, 17*(1), 149–174.

[8] ABC News. (2020, April 3). *Competition among state, local governments creates bidding war for medical equipment*. https://abcnews.go.com/US/competition-state-local-governments-creates-bidding-war-medical/story?id=69961539

[9] *Agit-prop* is shorthand for "agitational-propaganda" film, a type of documentary in which the filmmakers take a distinctive political or cultural position on an issue and are not particularly interested in showing what others might think, except to debunk those that oppose their views.

[10] Chillag, K. (2020, March 18). Social distancing cinema: A curated guide to epidemic movies. *Davidson College News*. https://www.davidson.edu/news/2020/03/18/social-distancing-cinema-curated-guide-epidemic-movies

13. Behave as if You Are Contagious (Health Economics)

[1] The theory of perfect competition can be traced to the writing of French economist Léon Walras, who gave the first rigorous definition of perfect competition and derived some of its main results. See Walras, L. (1954). *Elements of pure economics, or the theory of social wealth* (W. Jaffé, Trans.). Allen & Unwin. (Original work published 1874.) In the 1950s, U.S. economist Kenneth Arrow and French economist Gérard Debreu refined the theory in Arrow, K. J., & Debreu, G. (1954). Existence of an equilibrium for a competitive economy. *Econometrica, 22*(3), 265.

[2] Markets can never achieve perfect competition because the conditions together satisfy an abstract theoretical model.

[3] Obviously, people go to the doctor with various outcomes in mind. Some people do know what they want as an outcome (e.g., a prescription they have seen in an advertisement); others go simply seeking relief because they do not feel well.

[4] Many consumers fear financial risk from unexpectedly falling ill or becoming injured, even when they have health insurance. Seventy-nine million Americans are struggling to pay medical bills or have medical-related debt. Those without adequate health insurance risk health and financial ruin. See the Commonwealth Fund. (n.d.). *Survey: 79 million Americans have problems with medical bills or debt*. https://www.commonwealthfund.org/publications/newsletter-article/survey-79-million-americans-have-problems-medical-bills-or-debt

[5] There are also positive externalities. For example, if no one in your family smokes, you benefit. The concept of externalities requires us to think about both individual choice and societal well-being.

[6] Approximately 18% of those infected do not exhibit symptoms. See Mizumoto, K., Kagaya, K., Zarebski, A., & Chowell, G. (2020). Estimating the asymptomatic proportion of coronavirus disease 2019 (COVID-19) cases on board the Diamond Princess cruise ship, Yokohama, Japan, 2020. *Eurosurveillance, 25*(10). https://doi.org/10.2807/1560-7917.ES.2020.25.10.2000180

14. Discover a Blueprint to See a Way Out (History)

[1] Historians simply cannot know how a pandemic will play out, and they would not dare, in good conscience, make fortune-telling predictions. Taking time to observe, gather objective evidence, and reflect are all necessary before making any assessments concerning human or government (local, national, and international) responses to counter the spread of this new virus.

[2] These statistics come from a number of sources: Jernigan, D. B. (2018, May 4). *100 years since 1918: Are we ready for the next pandemic?* [PowerPoint slides]. Centers for Disease Control and Prevention. https://www.cdc.gov/flu/pandemic-resources/1918-commemoration/pdfs/1918-pandemic-webinar.pdf. The statistics for SARS (2017, December 6) are from https://www.cdc.gov/sars/; for MERS (2019, August 2), from https://www.cdc.gov/coronavirus/mers/index.html; for Ebola (2019, November 5), from https://www.cdc.gov/vhf/ebola/index.html; and for H1N1, 1918–1920, from the Centers for Disease Control and Prevention, 1918 Pandemic Flu Partner Webinar. The statistics for HIV/AIDS are from the Centers for Disease Control and Prevention. (2020, June 25). *HIV/AIDS basic statistics*. https://www.cdc.gov/hiv/basics/statistics.html. The statistics for malaria are from the Centers for Disease Control and Prevention. (2019, August 15). *Fighting the world's deadliest animal*. https://www.cdc.gov/globalhealth/stories/world-deadliest-animal.html

[3] Worldometer. *COVID-19 coronavirus pandemic*. https://www.worldometers.info/coronavirus/?utm_campaign=homeAdUOA?Si

[4] Mark, J. J. (2020, April 3). Boccaccio on the Black Death: Text & commentary. *Ancient History Encyclopedia*. https://www.ancient.eu/article/1537/boccaccio-on-the-black-death-text--commentary/

[5] The bat is feared because it has been linked to the emergence of several viral diseases (SARS, MERS, and COVID-19). But David Schneider, a disease ecologist at Stanford University, puts another spin on the bat: "Rather than vilifying bats, perhaps humans should consider them our allies in the fight against disease. I always hope, you know, how can we become more bat-like? That's the way to do it." See Wu, K. J. (2020,

May 5). *COVID-19 reignites a contentious debate over bats and disease*. Undark. https://undark.org/2020/05/05/covid-19-bats/

[6] *The Decameron*, completed in 1353, consists of 100 fictional stories written by 10 fictional narrators. The stories are comedic—they still have the power to bring laughter 667 years later—and sensual. Every social stratum is lampooned: from peasants to priests, from nobility to merchants. And men and women are made the butt of jokes equally. Humor and mortality can be great levelers. No one escaped Boccaccio's gaze, a fact that mirrors all too well the Black Death that did not discriminate. The Black Death affected people in all walks of life. Boccaccio's 10 fictional narrators were as cognizant of the plague as those who faced it in the "real" world. This attribute adds a dose of stark realism to his text; he masterfully managed to capture a horrific moment in human history. Boccaccio placed the narrators within 10 days of storytelling, in a country villa to which they had fled from Florence to outlast the plague and to distract themselves with bawdy tales. Each tale, titled by day and story number, begins with a short heading explaining the plot of the story. Boccaccio, G. (1353). *The Decameron of Giovanni Boccaccio* (J. M. Rigg, Trans.). Privately printed. https://publicdomainreview.org/collection/the-decameron

15. Know How Your Information Is Being Shared (Informatics)

[1] This suggests that, as part of a broader liberal arts education, studying the informatics fields could open the doors to careers that are in some sense "crisis-ready," careers that are less at risk of being interrupted by a pandemic, and, perhaps, assist society in responding to such crises.

[2] O'Neill, P. H., Ryan-Mosley, T., & Johnson, B. (2020, May 7). A flood of coronavirus apps are tracking us. Now it's time to keep track of them. *MIT Technology Review*. https://www.technologyreview.com/2020/05/07/1000961/launching-mittr-covid-tracing-tracker/

[3] Google. (2020, May 7). *Exposure notification: Frequently asked questions*. https://blog.google/documents/73/Exposure_Notification_-_FAQ_v1.1.pdf

16. Turn to Mathematics to Know How We Are Doing (Mathematics)

[1] To be clear, when I use the word "problem-solving," I am not referring to solving the kind of problems you typically find in a mathematics textbook.

[2] Before coming up with this question, I discarded several "unanswerable" questions, such as "Is the social and economic cost of social distancing worth the health benefits?" This question is overwhelming because there are so many costs—costs that vary widely by person—to consider. Also, many people report gains from social distancing.

[3] This team of researchers took on this challenge and "dropped everything they were doing to work on this around the clock." See Lempinen, E. (2020, June 8). Emergency COVID-19 measures prevented more than 500 million infections, study finds. *Berkeley News.* https://news.berkeley.edu/2020/06/08/emergency-covid-19-measures-prevented-more-than-500-million-infections-study-finds/

[4] Global Policy Lab. (2020). *The effect of large-scale anti-contagion policies on the COVID-19 pandemic.* http://www.globalpolicy.science/covid19#code-and-data

[5] The researchers found that the rates of infection were increasing by an average of about 38% per day when lockdowns began going into effect.

17. Support the Artists You Turn to in Times of Crisis (Music)

[1] Montagu, J. (2017, June 20). *Frontiers in Sociology, 2,* 8.

[2] Karadag, E., Uğur, Ö., & Çetinayak, O. (2019). The effect of music listening intervention applied during radiation therapy on the anxiety and comfort level in women with early-stage breast cancer: A randomized controlled trial. *European Journal of Integrative Medicine, 27,* 39–44. See also Çelebi, D., Yılmaz, E., Şahin, S. T., & Baydur, H. (2020, February). The effect of music therapy during colonoscopy on pain, anxiety and patient comfort: A randomized controlled trial. *Complementary Therapies in Clinical Practice,* 38. See also Çiftçi, H., & Öztunç, G. (2015, September–December). The effect of music on comfort, anxiety and pain in the Intensive Care Unit: A case in Turkey. *International Journal of Caring Sciences, 8*(3), 594–603.

[3] See Trevarthen, C., & Malloch, S. (2000) The dance of wellbeing: Defining the musical therapeutic effect. *Nordic Journal of Music Therapy, 9*(2), 3–17. https://doi.org/10.1080/08098130009477996. See also Malloch, S., & Trevarthen, C. (2018, October 4). The human nature of music. *Frontiers in Psychology, 9,* 1680. https://doi.org/10.3389/fpsyg.2018.01680.

[4] McCaffrey, R. (2008). Music listening: Its effects in creating a healing environment. *Journal of Psychosocial Nursing and Mental Health Services, 46*(10), 39–44. https://doi.org/10.3928/02793695-20081001-08

[5] Perryman, K., Blisard, P., & Moss, R. (2019, January). Using creative arts in trauma therapy: The neuroscience of healing. *Journal of Mental Health Counseling, (41)*1, 80–94.

[6] For the Record. (2020, March 3). *How social distancing has shifted Spotify streaming.* Spotify. https://newsroom.spotify.com/2020-03-30/how-social-distancing-has-shifted-spotify-streaming/

[7] Hissong, S. (2020, April 7). "Hey Siri, play songs to calm me down." What the world is listening to amid COVID-19. *Rolling Stone.* https://www.rollingstone.com/pro/news/streaming-moods-genres-coronavirus-979334/

[8] Hall, S. (2020, May 27). *This is how COVID-19 is affecting the music industry.* World Economic Forum. https://www.weforum.org/agenda/2020/05/this-is-how-covid-19-is-affecting-the-music-industry/

[9] Shaw, L. (2020, June 9). *This is one genre of music that isn't hurting right now.* Bloomberg. https://www.bloomberg.com/graphics/pop-star-ranking/2020-june/this-is-one-genre-of-music-that-isn-t-hurting-right-now.html

[10] Live performances by those who perform in close proximity (such as choruses and choirs) will certainly have to be rethought in the context of the coronavirus. See Hamner, L., Dubbel, P., Capron, I., Ross, A., Jordan, A., Lee, J., Lynn, J., Ball, A., Narwal, S., Russell, S., Patrick, D., & Leibrand, H. (2020, May 15). High SARS-CoV-2 attack rate following exposure at a choir practice—Skagit County, Washington. *MMWR Morbidity and Mortality Weekly Report 2020, 69,* 606–610. http://dx.doi.org/10.15585/mmwr.mm6919e6

[11] Some organizations have tried to pay their artists at least a portion of the fee they would have earned for cancelled performances. These payments are often made via donors who know the artists and want to provide active support. This has been a lifeline for many, but these payments can also prevent full unemployment benefits from being claimed by musicians. See Finkelstein, Z. (2020, April 8). The new heroes of COVID-19: 179 organizations who paid artists and counting . . . *The Middleclass Artist.* www.middleclassartist.com/post/the-new-heroes-of-covid-19-179-organizations-who-paid-artists-and-counting

18. Understand That Crises Can Be Managed (Organizational Leadership)

[1] Johnson, C. E. (2019). *Meeting the ethical challenges of leadership: Casting light or shadow.* SAGE.

[2] Johnson, C. E. (2019). *Meeting the ethical challenges of leadership: Casting light or shadow*. SAGE.

[3] Bazerman, M. H., & Watkins, M. D. (2004). *Predictable surprises: The disasters you should have seen coming, and how to prevent them*. Harvard Business School Press.

19. Stand Up for the Marginalized and Vulnerable (Philosophy)

[1] Samuels, A. (2020, April 21). Dan Patrick says, "There are more important things than living and that's saving this country." *Texas Tribune*. https://www.texastribune.org/2020/04/21/texas-dan-patrick-economy-coronavirus/

[2] Frimpong-Mansoh, A. (2008). Culture and voluntary informed consent in African health care systems. *Developing World Bioethics, 8*(2), 104–114.

[3] Rawls, J. A. (1999). *Theory of justice* (Rev. ed.). Harvard University Press. (Original work published 1971)

[4] Lahut, J. (2020, April 7). Fauci says the coronavirus is "shining a bright light" on "unacceptable" health disparities for African Americans. *Business Insider*. https://www.businessinsider.com/fauci-covid-19-shows-unacceptable-disparities-for-african-americans-2020-4

20. Join Together in an Age of Apart (Political Science)

[1] This includes governance at local, county, state, national, and international levels.

[2] Alexis de Tocqueville (1835) provided tremendous insight around the development of early American democracy. He touches on the importance of associations throughout his text, noting that "governments, therefore, should not be the only active powers; associations ought, in democratic nations, to stand in lieu of those powerful private individuals whom the equality of conditions has swept away." He goes on to describe the tradition of associations in America: "As soon as several of the inhabitants of the United States have taken up an opinion or a feeling which they wish to promote in the world, they look out for mutual assistance; and as soon as they have found one another out, they combine. From that moment they are no longer isolated men, but a power seen from afar, whose actions serve for an example and whose language is listened to." See Tocqueville, A. de. (1835). *Democracy in America*. Vintage Classics.

[3] Groups also maintain democracy by influencing public policy, the process by which local, state, and federal governments translate political vision into policies (e.g., on issues related to abortion, education, gun control, and social security). In policy making, it is important that all the parties affected by them are represented. In the absence of people-centered associations, the policy making process becomes imbalanced to the advantage of elites and the interest groups they dominate.

[4] To see how much of your life is regulated by local laws known as ordinances, look up the list of ordinances that govern the city or county where you live. Two examples of local ordinances are (1) "It shall be unlawful for any person to live in any boat, automobile, camper, mobile home, truck, or other motor vehicle within the limits of the city except for mobile homes located within the appropriate zone of the city" (Ordinance 83-0602, Campbell County, Kentucky) and (2) "It shall be unlawful for any person in any park to sleep in a prone position on the seats, tables or benches." Forest City, North Carolina, Code of Ordinances (Article I Section 15-7).

[5] Other examples of associations are Rotary clubs (bring together business and professional leaders in humanitarian service) and Kiwanis International clubs (serve the needs of children through local service projects).

[6] From Teorell, J. (2003). Linking social capital to political participation: Voluntary associations and networks of recruitment in Sweden. *Scandinavian Political Studies, 26*(1), 49–66.

[7] Snow, D. A., & Soule, S. A. (2010). *A primer on social movements*. W. W. Norton.

[8] The demonstrations that have occurred since George Floyd's death are unique because, unlike previous Black Lives Matter protests, these have been more sustained in nature (e.g., some protestors have camped outside City Hall in New York City for long periods of time, waiting for a change on police funding), they have occurred in all 50 states, and they have taken place even in small towns and in rural settings. The protests are also multigenerational. Finally, the speed at which things are changing (e.g., statues removed, cities renamed) as a result of the demonstrations is remarkable.

[9] Other rallies since the onset of the pandemic include the Supreme Court's ruling extending employment protections based on sex to the LGBTQ+ community so that gender and sexuality are also protected and President Trump's political campaign rallies. For those present at each event, it is clear that "the people" could not wait for the pandemic to end.

[10] The activities listed fall under the umbrella of "placemaking." Lydon and Garcia (2015) provide excellent

examples of a specific type of placemaking termed *tactical urbanism*. Tactical urbanism includes low-cost, temporary changes to the built environment, usually in cities, intended to improve local neighborhoods and city gathering places. Tactical urbanism is also commonly referred to as guerrilla urbanism, pop-up urbanism, city repair, or DIY urbanism. See Lydon, M., & Garcia, A. (2015). *Tactical urbanism: Short-term action for long-term change.* Island Press.

21. Imagine How the Pandemic Affects Everyone Across the Lifespan (Psychological Science)

[1] Schaie, K. W. (1986). Beyond calendar definitions of age, time, and cohort: The general developmental model revisited. *Developmental Review, 6*(3), 252–277.

[2] Baltes, P. B., Reese, H. W., & Lipsitt, L. P. (1980). Life span developmental psychology. *Annual Review of Psychology, 31,* 65–110.

[3] Other factors intersect with age to affect reactions and responses to crisis, including gender, race/ethnicity, sexual orientation, and disability status.

[4] Atypical events, such as a teenager losing their mother to death, might mean the teenager takes on the responsibilities and maturity of someone much older (becoming the mother figure for younger siblings) and foregoes the more typical expectations for youth.

[5] This idea of adapting to the changes a crisis brings to our lives can be difficult because this is when we most crave consistency, routine, and familiarity. The need for constancy is demonstrated in how our brains resist contrary information and how easily our actions become habits.

[6] "Coming of age" refers to a time during which people leave childhood and are moving toward adulthood. Beliefs about when children come of age vary across cultures. In the United States, people are legally considered children until they reach the age of 18.

22. Keep Looking for the Students Who Have Not Connected (School Counseling)

[1] U.S. Bureau of Labor Statistics. (2020, April 10). School and career counselors. *Occupational Outlook Handbook.* https://www.bls.gov/ooh/community-and-social-service/school-and-career-counselors.htm

[2] Hussar, B., Zhang, J., Hein, S., Wang, K., Roberts, A., Cui, J., Smith, M., Bullock Mann, F., Barmer, A., & Dilig, R. (2020, May). *The condition of education.* National Center for Education Statistics at Institute of Education Sciences. https://nces.ed.gov/pubs2020/2020144.pdf

[3] Educators for Excellence. (2020, May). *Voices from virtual classrooms: Survey of America's educators on teaching during and after the COVID-19 outbreak.* https://e4e.org/voices-virtual-classroom

[4] Jones, R. (2020, May 22). Beaufort Co. schools haven't heard from 300+ students during coronavirus closure. Why? *The Island Packet.* https://www.islandpacket.com/news/local/education/article242898811.html

[5] The good news is that the rate in that Texas school district has decreased 27% from the first days and weeks after schools transitioned to virtual learning. Webb, S. (2020, May 11). Thousands of Houston-area students lose contact with schools during pandemic shutdown. *Houston Chronicle.* https://www.houstonchronicle.com/news/education/article/arae-students-school-missing-thousands-coronavirus-15261497.php

[6] While there have been significant challenges, there remains a notable portion of students who have thrived in this situation. My colleagues and I have observed students motivated to complete work on their own terms—often prior to due dates that had been established by their teachers. Some students appreciated having access to assignments that were posted for the week, and they were able to do the work early and have more free time for themselves.

24. Visualize Social Issues (Visual Arts)

[1] The field of visual arts has found ways to engage with the blind and visually impaired, encouraging touch using techniques such as 3D printing, embedding Braille into visual art, and adding texture and sound to paintings.

[2] A photograph's form has to do with the structure or shape of the image in relation to the rectangular frame that has captured it. The content is the basic thing itself that the camera has captured—whether it be a tree, or a lion, or a flower, or a house, or a hummingbird, or a person. It could be anything.

[3] Eliasson, O. (2016, January 18). *Why art has the power to change the world.* World Economic Forum. https://www.weforum.org/agenda/2016/01/why-art-has-the-power-to-change-the-world/

[4] I talked to (Greg) Clair Hoover and his wife, Ruth, at length. He told me, "I'm not proud of the fact that our milk is being sold. . . . I feel that the only reason it has

been sold throughout this whole period is that if they wouldn't take our milk it should be admitting there is something wrong in the area."

[5] Out of this experience, I created a book. It took one year to finish. That had seemed like a long time. See Del Tredici, R. (1980). *The people of Three Mile Island.* Sierra Club Books.

[6] In spite of its enormity, the full extent of the meltdown had been unexplored and underreported. Ambivalent language to describe anomalies rushed in where angels feared to tread; the meltdown was referred to as "transient"; the domestic terror of the situation was highjacked by professionals linking dire health problems to neurotic nuclear fear; and the commanding invisibility of the epic affair kept citizens suspended in a communications limbo. These trends returned, much enhanced, with the Chernobyl disaster in 1987 and the Fukushima Daiichi nuclear disaster in 2011.

[7] I wrote and put together a book of photographs and interviews documenting my experiences. Del Tredici, R. (1987). *At work in the fields of the bomb.* Harper & Row.

[8] I visited Semipalatinsk, Kurchatov City, Novaya Zemlya, Moscow, and Chelyabinsk.

[9] When I documented the bomb, I went to the fenced-in Trinity site in the Alamogordo Desert, where the first atomic bomb baptized the Earth in a fire that can never be put out. I went to the Hiroshima Peace Park on August 6, the anniversary of the day the United States dropped the first nuclear weapon on a living city (a 5-ton bomb on Hiroshima). I went to the pockmarked Nevada Test Site (now known as the Nevada National Security Site), where the Cold War lanced the Earth with 928 immortal explosions.

25. Learn How Another Culture Responds to Crises (World Languages)

[1] Thompson, D. (2020, May 6). What's behind South Korea's COVID-19 exceptionalism? *Atlantic Magazine.* https://www.theatlantic.com/ideas/archive/2020/05/whats-south-koreas-secret/611215/

[2] Koreans created phonebooth-like structures, which a patient enters and speaks through an intercom to hospital staff. If the medical staff needs to conduct a test, they reach into the booth through protected holes into arm-length gloves to swab the patient's nose and throat. The process takes about 7 minutes, and the staff clean the booth before the next patient enters. See Houser, K. (2020, March 23). *South Korea starts using "phone booths" for coronavirus tests.* Freethink. https://www.freethink.com/articles/coronavirus-tests

[3] Gallo, W. (2020, May 6). South Korea balances privacy, public health in virus fight. *Voice of America News.* https://www.voanews.com/east-asia-pacific/south-korea-balances-privacy-public-health-virus-fight

[4] KBS WORLD Radio. (2020, July 10). *Ex-pres. Park sentenced to 20 years in retrial for influence pedaling.* https://world.kbs.co.kr/service/news_view.htm?lang=e&Seq_Code=154768

[5] Like in the United States, myths about how to prevent COVID-19 are plentiful in South Korea. The myths reflect cultural beliefs and values about what makes one healthy.

Index

positive psychology, 14–15
privileged class, 5
psychological science, 82–86

Quarmmen, David, 50

racial categories
  Black, 26–28
  Hispanic, not considered, 108
  Native American, 24–26
  officially recognized in the United
    States, 24
  socially created, 108
radioactivity, 96, 97, 99
Rawls, John, 74–75
reader advocates, xvi–xvii
reading, xvi–xvii
resilience, 11, 12, 14, 15, 61, 83, 107
resilience-building therapies, 12–15
responses to trauma, 91

sages, xvi–xvii
Salzman, Ryan, 81
scapegoating, 3
school
  barriers to connecting, 88–90, 114
  college and universities, xiii
  counseling, 87–90
  enrollments, xiii
science, 8, 10, 61, 66, 69, 77, 82,
  86, 106
segregation, 23–24
social distancing
  benefits of, 53, 63
  as collective action, 53
  constraints on face-to-face, 77, 78, 79
  deeper meaning of, 23–28
  economic costs, 111
  ethical questions about, 73
  guidelines, xiii
  as an investment, 53
  mandates, 63
  meaning of, 63

physical distancing, 23
  quantifying, 63–64
  along racial lines, 23
  responses to, 92
  self-isolation, 20
social forces, 1, 105
sociology, 1–3
South Korean
  cultural assumptions, 102–103
  response to COVID-19, 102
  values, 103
stories
  dominant, 108
  emergent, 30–31, 108
  hegemonic, 29, 30, 108
  official, 30
  residual, 30
  sense-making tools, 13, 14, 29,
    30, 32, 89, 97
  significance, 29, 30, 32
strength-based therapy, 13
student philanthropy projects, 16–18
students
  absenteeism during COVID-19, 87
  connecting with, 87–90
  engaging with communities, 88–90
  majors and, xiii
  number enrolled in college, xiii
  playing sports, xiii
  reading during COVID-19, 39
sudden attentiveness, 19
Sugg, La Shanda, 94

Taylor, Breonna, 26, 31, 89
Taylor, Tedd, 98
thought experiments, 62, 64, 65
Three Mile Island, 96–97, 115
Time of Terror, 26
Tocqueville, Alexis de, 113
"together apart," 59
Transtromer, Thomas, 20–21
trauma
  coronavirus as global-scale trauma, 91

defined, 91
  faint response to 91, 92, 93
  finding "best" options in, 106
  flock response to, 9, 92, 93
  freeze response, 91, 92, 93
  human survival responses to, 93
  manage response to, 67
  music as a response to, 112
  therapies, 11–15, 67, 112
trauma studies, 91–94
trust in ideas, 3, 7, 10, 15, 18, 22,
  28, 32, 36, 40, 45, 53, 58, 61,
  65, 69, 72, 76, 81, 86, 90, 94,
  100, 104

unanticipated consequences,
  2–3, 105
unemployment, 5, 13, 33, 49, 112
universal basic income, 31

veil of ignorance, 74–75
Vest, Jason, 69
visual arts, 95–100
vulnerable populations, 3, 9, 24–25,
  26, 50, 112, 113

Wallace, Robert K., 40
Weil, Simone, 21
well-being therapy, 12–13
White category
  extreme physical distancing
    and, 23–28
  "get out of our spaces," 28
  responses to racial injustice,
    27–28
world languages, 101

"X marks the spot" places, 96, 99

Zaniello, Tom, 50
Zembrodt, Isabella, 15
zoonotic virus transmission, 43,
  55, 109